American Medical Association
Physicians dedicated to the health of America

Starting
a Medical Practice
Second Edition

*Business Plans
SBA Loan.
Medical Management*

*Client Services @
Medical Mangement
. com*

Jeffery P. Daigrepont
The Coker Group

*720-951-8427
Fax 720-951 -
2157*

AMA press

Practice Success Series

Starting a Medical Practice
Second Edition

Internet address: www.ama-assn.org

This book is for informational purposes only. It is not intended to constitute legal or financial advice. If legal, financial, or other professional advice is required, the services of a competent professional should be sought.

Additional copies of this book may be ordered by calling 800 621-8335. Mention product number OP315202.

ISBN 1-57947-296-6

Library of Congress Cataloging-in-Publication Data

Daigrepont, Jeffery.
   Starting a medical practice / by Jeffery Daigrepont.— 2nd ed.

      p. ; cm. — (Practice success! series)
   Rev. ed. of: Starting a medical practice / Lauretta Mink. c1996.
   Includes bibliographical references and index.
   ISBN 1-57947-296-6 (alk. paper)
   1. Medicine—Practice.
   1. Practice Management, Medical—organization & administration—United States. 2. Facility Design and Construction—United States. 3. Professional Practice—legislation & jurisprudence—United States. W 80 D132s 2002: I. Mink, Lauretta. Starting a medical practice. II. American Medical Association. III. Title. IV. Series.

R728 .D25 2002
610'.68—dc21

                                                   2002151480

BQ13:02-P-47:03/03

The Coker Group, a leader in health care consulting, helps providers attain improved financial and operational results through sound business principles. The consulting team members are proficient, trustworthy professionals with experience and strengths in various areas. The well-rounded staff includes seasoned individuals in finance, administration, management, operations, compliance, personnel management, and information systems.

The Coker Group's nation-wide client base includes major health systems, hospitals, physician groups, and solo practitioners in a full spectrum of engagements. The Coker Group has gained a reputation since 1987 for thorough, efficient, and cost-conscious work to benefit its clients financially and operationally. The firm has a towering profile with recognized and respected health care professionals throughout the industry. Coker's exceptional consulting team has health care, technical, financial, and business knowledge and offers comprehensive programs, services, and training to yield long-term solutions and turnarounds. Coker staff members are devoted to delivering reliable answers and dependable options so that decision-makers can make categorical decisions. Coker consultants enable providers to concentrate on patient care.

Service Areas

- Practice management, billing and collection reviews, chart audits
- Procedural coding analysis
- Information systems review, including EMR
- Physician employment and compensation review
- Physician network development
- Practice appraisals
- Strategic planning/business planning
- Disengagements of practices and network unwinds
- Practice operational assessments
- Contract negotiations
- Hospital services, medical staff development
- Practice start-ups
- Buy/sell and equity analysis
- Sale/acquisition negotiations
- Group formation and dissolution
- Educational programs, workshops, and training
- Compliance plans
- HIPAA assessments and compliance

- MSA development
- Financial analysis
- Mediation and expert witnessing
- Policies and procedures manuals

For more information, contact:

The Coker Group
11660 Alpharetta Hwy / Suite 710 / Roswell, GA 30076
(800) 345.5829
www.cokergroup.com

Jeffery P. Daigrepont, a manager and shareholder of The Coker Group, specializes in practice start-ups, strategic planning, operations, and deployment of fully integrated information systems for the medical practice. Mr. Daigrepont focuses on the process of obtaining relevant data, converting it into useful information, and applying it to effective decision-making, which leads to operational improvements. Specifically, he is knowledgeable in EMR technology, patient privacy and security, HIPAA readiness, and optimizing practice revenue. He is a popular workshop speaker who addresses a variety of topics related to the management of the medical practice.

Mr. Daigrepont has a unique ability to interpret and communicate information in a meaningful way, enabling clients to fully understand the parameters of a situation and to arrive at a logical plan for reaching organizational goals and objectives.

Professional affiliations include *The Healthcare Information and Management Systems Society (HIMSS)*. HIMSS provides leadership in health care for the advancement and management of information technology. Mr. Daigrepont is in the process of attaining certification as a Professional in Healthcare Information and Management Systems (CPHIMS).

Additionally, Mr. Daigrepont is credentialed by *The American Academy of Medical Management* with an Executive Fellowship in Practice Management (EFMP) and as a Certified Administrator in Physician Practice Management (CAPPM). He also serves on the faculty of this organization as a workshop and seminar speaker.

By the time today's medical students complete their residencies and enter their chosen field, they will be in their early 30s, nearly $100,000 in debt, and facing administrative duties that would make their counterparts in the private sector balk, according to Julie Bryant, staff writer for the *Atlanta Business Chronicle*.[1]

Some physicians start out as employees in hopes of forgoing the headaches of management. They enter an existing practice that someone else has established years earlier or they become a part of a network of a large health system. However, these physicians, too, may at some future point find themselves thrust into start-up and management roles when they turn to independent practice—usually as a result of disengagement from the network.

Medical practice is a changing, challenging field. Physicians must spend much of their time wearing the hat of administrator in addition to engagement in an already complex profession. Being a physician will be a tougher row to hoe than a job in the private sector.

This book is about helping physicians start up a practice from a number of different points. Some will choose to become employees; some will join groups; some will become sole proprietors. Whether starting out at first or rebuilding after disengagement, the task is monumental. Many physicians who are leaving affiliations are working hard to regain the right to practice independently in their communities, and they symbolize a new movement in health care— the return of the independent practice.

The scope of starting a practice encompasses practice management, billing and collections, managed care, facility design, human resources, marketing, and purchasing. A practice start-up also includes selecting an office location and designing the practice space. It requires ordering all of the office and medical supplies and creating the practice's signage and marketing literature, and evaluating and selecting employee candidates. The details are endless.

Whether starting out fresh from a residency program or starting over in independent practice, this book will guide you through this difficult transition with a great deal of support, professionalism, and enthusiasm.

[1] Bryant, Julie, "Passion for patient care, not dollars, guides new generation of physicians," *Atlanta Business Chronicle*. http://www.bizjournals.comindustries/health_care/physicians_practices/2002/07/29/. 07/31/02.

CONTENTS

Getting Started

INTRODUCTION

The purpose of this chapter is to set forth the processes for formulating your decision to establish your medical practice and to direct you to the appropriate resources necessary to help you get off to a good start. By strategically mapping out an action plan organized in a timeline from beginning to end, you will be able to approach this initiative systematically and in accord with your goals and desired results.

FACTORS INFLUENCING YOUR DECISION

Reaching the decision to start your own practices can evolve from a number of influencing factors depending on your goals, objectives, and, most importantly, your ambitions. The range of starting points will vary depending upon your personality, your unique circumstances, and the current phase of your professional career.

It is important to start organizing your decisions early and to allow plenty of time for adjustments or alternative considerations. Personal networking and professional advice is a wonderful way for you to obtain an inside prospective into what you may be considering and for what to expect. At the beginning of this initiative, a number of influencing factors will exist, but none will be more vital than your personal aspirations and desires for success. Table 1-1 is a decision-making tool to help with the process.

How Did You Score?

After answering the questions in Table 1-1, which column contained the highest score?

- **Sole Proprietor.** If you scored the highest in the sole proprietor or solo practitioner column, you will likely be most comfortable as the principal/primary owner of your own medical practice. You may at some point, however, consider employing other physicians or mid-level providers. Furthermore, you may consider allowing a partner to buy into the practice at some point; you will likely always want to maintain for yourself the position of majority shareholder.

TABLE 1-1

Practice Style Decision-Maker

(Circle the answer that applies.)

Questions	Sole Proprietor	Partnership or Group Practice— Part-Owner	Employed
1. Do you prefer to make your own decisions?	Yes	Somewhat	No
2. Are you comfortable with making difficult decisions?	Yes	Somewhat	No
3. Are you organized and detailed oriented?	Yes	Somewhat	No
4. Do you perform well under productivity incentives to see X number of patients?	No	Somewhat	Yes
5. Do you perform well when having your clinical utilization monitored?	No	Somewhat	Yes
6. Do you enjoy marketing and networking?	Yes	Somewhat	No
7. Are you willing to compromise on your objectives or settle on an issue?	No	Somewhat	Yes
8. Are you a competent record keeper?	Yes	Somewhat	No
9. Do you enjoy managing and leadership?	Yes	Somewhat	No
10. Are you good at containing expenses?	Yes	Somewhat	No
11. Do you have the mindset of a business owner who can focus on profits, in addition to patient care?	Yes	Somewhat	No
TOTAL:			

- **Partnership or Group Practice.** Always a good starting point to test comfort level with running your own practice, a partnership or group practice will enable you to experience the environment and share the responsibility with your colleagues. In order to have a positive experience in joining a group or partnership, it is important that you fully understand the culture, its leadership, its goals, and your personal responsibility within the group. Moreover, take time to fully understand your contract, especially the out-clause provisions and the non-compete provisions.

- **Employed.** If you scored highest in the employed column, it does not necessarily mean that owning your own practice is not a viable option for you. Many successful solo practitioners started off as employed physicians with full intentions of starting their own practice in a year or two. Starting off as an employed physician provides exposure to how a medical practice operates, and it will give you some time to save money for a sole proprietorship. Also, successful solo practitioners exist who are in private practice who did not first become employed, but as an alternative they engaged the experience and assistance of professionals to help start their practice.

No single approach is right for every physician—it's a matter of personal preference. However, every physician starting out in practice shares the common objective to be successful. The focus of this chapter is to begin thinking about the decisions when starting your own practice. Various options, such as employment, group practices, partnerships, and practice structures, are addressed in Chapter 2, *Choosing an Organizational Structure.*

Next we will explore the factors and decisions for determining the success of a medical practice.

Helping Ensure Your Success

Knowing where you are needed and, more importantly, knowing exactly how to position your practice within that community can determine whether or not you will be successful. There are several factors to consider when choosing a practice's location.

- **Professional Relationships and Opportunities.** Professional relationships include those that were formed during medical school and those with practicing physicians who have influenced your career. Professional opportunities encompass what an area presents for continuing education, professional stimulation, and the opportunity to practice in a hospital offering the most advanced technology and facilities. Also, you will want to consider whether the area provides opportunities for professional growth for your spouse.

- **Prior Exposure.** Where you went to medical school, your residency program location, and your place of birth may all influence your choice of location. Nearly 50 percent of physicians who practice in towns with populations less than 2,500 grew up in towns of similar size. Studies suggest that there is also a strong relationship between location of postgraduate training and the location of a private practice.

- **Economic Factors.** Salary or income potential and cost of living are also strong determinants in the choice of geographical location. Before choosing a location, determine if the area in question is an area of need, in a depressed economy, or in an area of rapid growth. Depending on your specialty, you should learn whether the growth in the area is due to an influx of young families or is the result of a booming retirement community.

Small towns where the community is medically under served often provide opportunities for the highest income. Research the demographics of the location for population, the per capita income, age, and gender mix.

Your personality and your specialty are the underlying factors for whether you would be content to establish your practice in a rural or underserved area. Although 20 percent of the US population lives in rural areas, only 9 percent of physicians practice there, and only 3 percent of recent medical school graduates plan to do so. Most rural physicians are generalists, while family physicians are the only specialty group that distributes itself proportionally to the population in rural and urban areas.[1]

- **Environmental Factors.** Quality and availability of housing, cultural opportunities, and the educational system should all be considered when selecting a location. Proximity to a major airport, public transportation, and recreational opportunities

---

[1] Health leaders fact file. *Journal of the American Medical Association.* http://www.healthleaders.com/magazine/print.php?contentid=37158&section=factfile. 09/04/02.

will also influence your decision. Finally, climate and even pollution may be factors to consider.

■ **Other Determinants.** Hospital proximity, religious affiliations, group practice opportunities, and the availability of other physicians are important. The new physician entering solo practice will also want to check availability and average cost per square foot for office space.

Take the time to write down your objectives, constraints, and goals for success. Use those goals and objectives to help you in the decision-making process. Many sources are available for obtaining information about practice opportunities in geographic locations that best suit your needs.

Where to Look for Employment Opportunities

The following is a brief list of places to look for employment opportunities:

■ Residency Program Directors
■ American Medical Association's placement service
■ Specialty Society placement service
■ State and County medical societies
■ Classified ads in journals (eg, *Journal of the American Medical Association, New England Journal of Medicine,* and specialty journals)

Where to Find Information Concerning a Geographic Location

When in need of specific geographic location information, the following are great sources:

■ Regional Planning Commission
■ Census Bureau (Local offices are available in major cities and state capitals. Be specific about the information that is needed.)
■ State Department of Tourism
■ Area Chamber of Commerce
■ Local and state medical societies

How to Determine the Area's Need for a Physician

When searching for a practice location, the following will help in determining an area in need:

■ County or state medical society
■ Chief of Staff at the area hospital(s)
■ Other physicians
■ Pharmacists

- Local health systems agency (if available) can provide critical information about physician demographics, hospital beds, occupancy rates, underserved areas, and other health care delivery systems, such as ambulatory care centers, family planning clinics, and physician extenders.
- Sunday newspapers from the areas under consideration. It may be wise to subscribe or arrange to purchase these routinely.

Once the options have been narrowed to two or three locations, visit these areas at least once before making a final selection. Visit the local hospitals and talk with the Chiefs of Staff. Determine how long it will take to obtain hospital privileges. Make sure the hospital(s) is not closed to new staff members.

If you are planning to open a practice of your own, you will need at least 12 months lead time to do your research, select a location, and complete other necessary arrangements. Because so many details are involved, a time line is provided to help you stay on track (Table 1-2). The Location Decision Scorecard (Table 1-3) can be used to rate and compare the professional, economic, and residential characteristic of potential practice sites. Using these tools will ensure awareness of everything that must be accomplished before joining a group or opening your own practice.

TABLE 1-2

Time Line for Starting to Practice Medicine

Photocopy this time line and keep it as a reference. Work on completing these steps whenever possible.

Not all requirements will apply to all practice options. We have coded each line:

E = Employed physician

GP = Physicians joining a group practice

SP = Physician starting a solo private practice

One Year before Starting Practice

		Check as completed	Responsible party
1.	Make final decision on practice location. (E, GP, SP)	❐	_____
2.	Check on membership for: (E, GP, SP)		
	County medical society	❐	_____
	State medical society	❐	_____
	American Medical Association	❐	_____
	Specialty society	❐	_____
3.	For comparison purposes, get the details in writing of contracts from groups or corporations that are being considered (GP, E). (See group practice questionnaire in Chapter 3, Selecting Your Professional Path.)	❐	_____
4.	Begin to examine net worth in terms of capital available for start-up costs. (SP) (See Chapter 9, Financing the Medical Practice.)	❐	_____
5.	If possible, reserve office telephone number (or answering service number). (SP)	❐	_____
6.	Find out the date when telephone books are printed. Have the practice name listed in both the white and yellow pages. (SP)	❐	_____

TABLE 1-2 *Continued*

	Check as completed	Responsible party
7. Visit banks and begin shopping for a loan. Pick up loan applications and meet loan officers. Determine what information the bank will need to evaluate the loan application. (SP) (See Chapter 9, Financing the Medical Practice.)	☐	_____
8. Open:		
Checking account, personal (E, GP, SP)	☐	_____
Checking account, business (SP)	☐	_____
Savings account, personal (E, GP, SP)	☐	_____
Savings account, business (SP)	☐	_____
9. Draw up an income/expenditure projection for first year of practice. Talk with several bankers regarding borrowing money; submit applications. (SP) (See Chapter 9, Financing the Medical Practice.)	☐	_____

Nine Months before Starting Practice

1. Check sites for leasing/buying medical office space. (SP)	☐	_____
2. Check zoning ordinances with local city hall and/or zoning board regarding signage, type of businesses allowed in the area; ask about any anticipated changes. (SP)	☐	_____
3. Check on utility requirements for the office. (SP)	☐	_____
4. If leasing, see if any leasehold improvements are needed and when these improvements can be made. (SP) (See Chapter 10, Selecting and Leasing Space and Purchasing Equipment.)	☐	_____
5. Determine office layout and design. (SP)	☐	_____
6. Determine office and medical equipment needed. If installing x-ray equipment, check with the state health department, radiological health section, to see if they require special registration or certification. Make the same checks for laboratory or outpatient surgery facilities. (SP) (For laboratory license information, see Chapter 4, Regulations and Licensing Requirements.)	☐	_____
7. Choose advisors (as appropriate). (See Chapter 1, Getting Started.)		
Accountant (E, GP, SP)	☐	_____
Attorney (E, GP, SP)	☐	_____
Banker (E, GP, SP)	☐	_____
Insurance broker(s) (E, GP, SP)	☐	_____
Management consultant (SP)	☐	_____
Real estate broker (E, GP, SP)	☐	_____
Other (eg, computer consultant) (E, GP, SP)	☐	_____
8. Evaluate office lease and/or partnership agreement contracts with an attorney before signing them. (See Chapters 3, Selecting a Professional Path, and 10, Selecting and Leasing Space and Purchasing Equipment.)	☐	_____
9. Obtain bids on major office equipment that will be needed; compare leasing versus purchasing. Be sure to get a written guarantee of delivery date and in-transit insurance. (See equipment list and budget in Chapter 10, Selecting and Leasing Space and Purchasing Equipment.)		
Select a practice management system (SP) Standalone system, Application Service Provider	☐	_____
Consider electronic medical records (SP)	☐	_____
Consider billing options (eg, in-house, outsource) (SP)	☐	_____
Dictation equipment (SP) (N/A with EMR)	☐	_____
Intercom system (ie, determine whether it will be separate from telephones) (SP)	☐	_____
Exam room/medical equipment (SP)	☐	_____
Photocopy machine (SP)	☐	_____
Computer/typewriter/word processor (SP)	☐	_____
Telephone equipment (SP)	☐	_____

T A B L E 1-2 *Continued*

	Check as completed	Responsible party
Calculator (SP)	☐	_____
Light signaling system (SP)	☐	_____
Reception room/office furniture and decorations (SP)	☐	_____
Tool kit/flashlight (SP)	☐	_____
10. If in a partnership, complete the details of the partnership agreement; have it drawn up and signed by each partner.	☑	_____
11. Obtain narcotics license: (E, GP, SP)		
Federal: Application for registration available through the Department of Justice, Drug Enforcement Administration, local or state office. If necessary, contact the national office: Drug Enforcement Administration, P.O. Box 28083, Central Station, Washington, DC 20005, (202) 724-1013.	☑	_____
State: Check local medical licensing board to see who issues licenses in the state. The state pharmacy board or the Department of Registration and Education usually does this.	☐	_____
12. Inform the state medical licensing board of the new address. (E, GP, SP)	☐	_____

Six Months before Starting Practice

	Check as completed	Responsible party
1. Obtain the services of an answering service: (SP)		
Physicians' exchange (eg, hospital or medical society) (E, SP, GP)		
Personal (office) (SP)	☐	_____
Beeper service (SP)	☐	_____
Call-forwarding (SP)	☐	_____
2. Select a Pension Plan or Individual Retirement Account.	☐	_____
3. Check with the medical society regarding their position and guidelines on advertising in the local newspaper, and other forms of announcements. Many will provide mailing labels and assist with printing. (SP)	☑	_____
4. Meet with the professional representative from the Medicare fiscal intermediary (the local medical society will offer advice on this), Medicaid administered by the state health and human services agency, and major commercial carriers regarding: (See Chapter 4, Regulations and Licensing Requirements.)		
Provider number(s) (SP, E, GP, check with employer)	☐	_____
Medicare fee schedule (SP)	☐	_____
5. Obtain a Current Procedural Terminology book (CPT-4). (SP)	☐	_____
6. Obtain an International Classification of Diseases Book (ICD-9-CM). (SP)	☐	_____
7. Apply for hospital staff privileges. (SP, E, GP)	☑	_____
8. Arrange to attend Grand Rounds at the local hospital(s). (SP, E, GP)	☐	_____
9. Order medical record system. (SP) (N/A with EMR)	☐	_____
10. Order sign for office. (SP)	☐	_____
11. Order insurance forms (HCFA 1500 Claim Form from the AMA: 800 621-8335).	☐	_____
12. Notify pharmaceutical representatives and other appropriate salespersons of the new practice.	☐	_____
13. Obtain county and city occupational licenses available from the county/city clerk's office or city hall. (See Chapter 4, Regulations and Licensing Requirements.)	☐	_____

Three Months before Starting Practice

	Check as completed	Responsible party
1. Arrange for professional malpractice insurance. (SP, GP, E; check with employer).	☐	_____
2. Arrange for office insurance. (Call 800 458-5736 for information on AMA-sponsored insurance plan.) (SP) (See Chapter 8, Identifying Insurance Requirements.)	☐	_____
Office overhead (SP)	☐	_____
Office liability (SP)	☐	_____

TABLE 1-2 *Continued*

	Check as completed	Responsible party
Business interruption (SP)	☐	_____
Employee fidelity bond (SP)	☐	_____
Office contents (SP)	☐	_____
Umbrella: Provides comprehensive catastrophic liability coverage for liability claims beyond the limits of regular liability programs. (SP)	☐	_____
Workers' Compensation: This is often required by law and is determined on a state-by-state basis. Check with the state's workers' compensation board or industrial commission. (SP)	☐	_____
Health: Major medical for self, dependents, and employees.	☐	_____
Disability (SP, E, GP; check with employer)	☐	_____
Life (SP, E, GP)	☐	_____
Automobile (SP, E, GP)	☐	_____

3. Arrange for telephone service installation. Consider purchasing telephone equipment. (SP) ☐ _____

4. Consider a money market fund, opened directly or with the bank. (SP) ☐ _____

5. Consider arranging for acceptance of credit cards (eg, VISA, MasterCard American Express) at the new office through a local bank. (Call 800-366-6968 for information on AMA-sponsored VISA program.) (SP) ☐ _____

6. Talk with the local newspaper regarding practice announcement ads. ☐ _____

7. Order office-opening announcements. ☐ _____

8. Arrange to give talks to community groups on health topics. (SP, GP) (See Chapter 15, Building the Practice through Marketing.) ☐ _____

9. Meet physicians who are potential referral sources. Send letters, arrange appointments. (SP, GP) ☐ _____

10. Find out if a patient referral service is available through the local medical society. Send them essential information. (SP, GP) ☐ _____

11. Check on memberships in civic and church organizations. (SP, E, GP) ☐ _____

12. Arrange for movers, if necessary. (SP, E, GP) ☐ _____

13. Write to the State Department of Labor for state employment regulations and Wage and Hour information. (SP) ☐ _____

14. Write preliminary job descriptions for employees. (SP) ☐ _____

15. Write policy manual for office employees. (SP) ☐ _____

16. Check local resources for personnel. (SP) ☐ _____

17. Start interviewing for office/clinical personnel. (SP) ☐ _____

18. Apply for Federal Employer Identification Number through the local Internal Revenue Service Office (SS-4 Form). (SP) ☐ _____

19. Apply for State Employer Identification Number through the state employment office/labor department. (SP) ☐ _____

20. Obtain "Small Business Tax Guide" and Federal Estimated Income Tax Form through the local IRS office, or attend Small Business Tax Seminar at the local IRS office. (SP) ☐ _____

21. Write for State Estimated Income Tax Form through state department/labor department. (SP) ☐ _____

22. Obtain payroll-withholding booklets (ie, federal, state, city) through local IRS office. (SP) ☐ _____

23. Review tax requirements with accountant. (SP) ☐ _____

24. Plan and order appointment-scheduling book. (SP) ☐ _____

25. As needed, arrange for:

Janitorial service	☐	_____
Snow removal	☐	_____
Laundry service	☐	_____
Grounds maintenance	☐	_____

TABLE 1-2   *Continued*

		Check as completed	Responsible party
26.	Order clinical supplies and set-up inventory control system. (SP) (See Chapter 10, Selecting and Leasing Space and Purchasing Equipment.)	❐	_____
27.	Order business supplies: (SP)		
	Appointment cards	❐	_____
	Business cards	❐	_____
	Patient recall system	❐	_____
	Petty cash vouchers	❐	_____
	Letterhead stationery and envelopes	❐	_____
	Deposit stamp for checks	❐	_____
	Prescription pads	❐	_____
	Purchase order forms	❐	_____
	Preprinted telephone message pads	❐	_____
28.	Determine likely office hours based on community need. (SP) 8:30 → 5:00	❐	_____
29.	Determine fee schedule. (SP) — *Ched Simmont*	❐	_____
30.	Select and order magazines: (SP) — *Donations* *Saturday 8-12 p.*		
	For reception room	❐	_____
	Medical journals for self	❐	_____
31.	Purchase office equipment and furniture; arrange delivery date. (SP) *old furniture*	❐	_____
32.	Arrange for: (SP)		
	Laboratory services for patients	❐	_____
	X-ray services for patients	❐	_____
33.	Notify area pharmacies of new practice. (GP, SP)	❐	_____
34.	Write patient information booklet and have it printed. (SP) ✓ *Leaflet*	❐	_____

One Month before Starting Practice

		Check as completed	Responsible party
1.	Start setting up office. (SP)	❐	_____
2.	Have utilities tuned on:		
	Telephone	❐	_____
	Electricity	❐	_____
	Gas	❐	_____
	Water	❐	_____
3.	Start accepting appointments. (SP)	❐	_____
4.	Hire and train office personnel regarding: (SP)		
	Telephone techniques	❐	_____
	Collections	❐	_____
	Appointments	❐	_____
	Office policies	❐	_____
5.	Decide on collection/insurance policy. (SP)	❐	_____
6.	Hang out shingle (post sign). (SP)	❐	_____
7.	Establish a petty cash fund. (SP)	❐	_____
8.	Establish a charge fund. (SP)	❐	_____
9.	Place announcement in community paper and medical society bulletin: (SP, GP)		
	Advertisement	❐	_____
	News Release	❐	_____
10.	Mail out announcements to physicians, pharmacists, hospitals, and health groups. (SP, GP)	❐	_____
11.	Plan office "open house." (SP)	❐	_____

Opening Day of Practice

		Check as completed	Responsible party
1.	See first patient.	❐	_____
2.	Congratulate self. The practice is open!	❐	_____

T A B L E 1-3

Location Decision Scorecard

I. Rate a prospective location ten ways

Fill out one column for each area visited. Score: 5 = Yes, 3 = Doubtful, 0 = No.

		Communities	
	A	B	C
1. I'm convinced a need is here.			
2. The medical society was encouraging.			
3. Local doctors didn't dash my hopes.			
4. I can get hospital privileges.			
5. Coverage would be no problem.			
6. Consultation facilities are adequate.			
7. Postgraduate education is accessible.			
8. I can get suitable office space.			
9. Skilled office help is available.			
10. Key citizens think there is room for me.			
Totals			

II. Then, rate the economic prospects this way

Fill out one column for each area visited. Score: 5 = Yes, 3 = Doubtful, 0 = No.

		Communities	
	A	B	C
1. Population growing.			
2. Diversified industry.			
3. Good employment level.			
4. New firms moving in.			
5. Local bank debits rising.			
6. High wages.			
7. Low welfare rolls.			
8. Consumer credit good.			
9. Health insurance is popular.			
10. Going health care rates are acceptable.			
Totals			

III. Now, rate the residential prospects this way

Fill out one column for each area visited. Score: 5 = Yes, 3 = Doubtful, 0 = No.

		Communities	
	A	B	C
1. Spouse likes the place.			
2. Attractive residential section.			
3. Zoning laws guard property values.			
4. House prices within reach.			
5. Reasonable local taxes.			
6. Adequate public services.			
7. Plentiful shopping facilities.			
8. Good public school system.			
9. Adequate churches and cultural facilities.			
10. Adequate recreation facilities.			
Totals			

TABLE 1-3 *Continued*

IV. Finally, compare the towns' total scores

		Communities	
	A	B	C
Professional prospects.			
Economic prospects.			
Residential prospects.			
Totals			

Source: Reprinted with permission from American Academy of Pediatrics Committee on Practice and Ambulatory Medicine. *Management of Pediatric Practice*, 2nd ed., Elk Grove Village, IL, American Academy of Pediatrics, 1991:11.

You can delegate some objectives on the timetable to individuals that you trust. That person will need to be persistent and pay attention to detail. You, the physician, should take the responsibility of seeing that all the requirements are completed on time.

You will be asked to provide copies of all your licenses, identifier numbers, and other credentialing requirements several times. To prepare, begin now to build a file that includes the original and several copies of this information.

SELECTING PROFESSIONAL ASSISTANCE

Because of the complexity of business in general, and medical practice management, you cannot discount the need for professional advice and consultation. New physicians should trust their instincts and seek guidance from expert advisors, specifically professionals experienced in health care. To help you through the complex maze of professional advisors, the following are summaries of their services and the roles they are expected to play. It may be wise to seek recommendations from other physicians concerning these advisors.

Legal Assistance

An attorney will help set up the legal structure of your practice or assist with reviewing your contract of employment or partnership. Only use attorneys who understand and have experience in health care law. They should also be considered for reviewing your lease, purchase agreements, and other contracts, especially those involving long-term commitments, such as a billing services agreement or practice management support contracts.

Accounting Assistance

To ensure that the practice provides the best tax advantages and flexibility, you will need to engage an experienced accountant. Along with the attorney, an accountant should be consulted before setting up your legal structure because the legal structure can affect tax advantages. The accountant will also assist with setting up accounting processes as well as establishing the internal controls for tracking cash flow, profit and loss statements, payroll withholdings, quarterly taxes, and operating budget. The person providing accounting advice does not necessarily have to be a Certified Public Accountant (CPA). Nonetheless, selecting the right accountant should be considered on the basis of technical knowledge and experience in health care and the ability to meet your needs. The following descriptions will help differentiate between the various types of accounting services.

- **Certified Public Accountant.** A CPA will typically have the highest level of expertise in the field of accounting due to their certification requirements. In addition, like other certified professionals, their field must comply with mandated regulations. A CPA will generally charge by the hour and is typically more expensive than other accounting services. Finding a CPA that is experienced in operations of medical practices will be well worth the extra investment.

- **Bookkeeping Services.** Bookkeeping services are widely available and can generally provide the same types of services as that of a CPA, but they may be limited in how much tax planning and/or business advice they can provide. Carefully check references and the reputation of bookkeeping firms that are being considered and, more significantly, verify that they are experienced in operations of medical practices.

- **Practice Management Services.** These companies generally assist with the full spectrum of operations. They can perform such services as hiring employees, maintaining the books, payroll, purchasing, billing and collections, managed care contracting, and other services related to operations. Their fees can be based on a percentage of net collections or a flat monthly fee. Typically the most common arrangement is to base fees on a percentage of net profits after expenses, so there is an incentive for both maximizing revenues and cost containment. It is important to verify references and, essentially, their success in managing operations of a medical practice.

- **Management Service Organizations (MSO).** An MSO is typically formed by hospitals that will allow its member to collectively share in benefits and services that are difficult to obtain on an individual basis. Such services include group purchasing, contracting with managed care, billing services, transcription, and staffing. The basic concept of an MSO is having strength in numbers. Because of Stark laws, an MSO owned by a hospital will rarely have any financial interest in a practice, and therefore they typically do not provide the accounting services or services related to the financial performance of the practice, as described in the other types of management services.

- **Independent Physician Organizations (IPO) or Independent Physician Associations (IPA).** These organizations can be similar to an MSO. However, they are generally seen in areas with a heavy concentration of managed care or capitation in the marketplace. Their primary focus is on obtaining market shares for its members as well as acceptable reimbursement from the payers. Most physicians who participate in these management organizations also maintain services with the professional services because IPOs and IPAs provide only a limited scope of services.

Regardless of whether you choose an accountant, bookkeeper, practice management services, or combine these services with an MSO, IPO, or IPA, be sure the service meets your needs, and do not underestimate your own ability to perform some services yourself. The following list contains services that could be considered for outsourcing:

- Establishing budgets and financial forecasting.
- Periodic reviews of the financial performance of the practice. This should include monthly preparation of financial statements.
- Routine audits, and checks and balances.
- Reconciliation of bank statements, deposits, credit card transactions, and accounts payable.
- Knowledge and consultative reviews of IRS laws and penalties.
- Consultative advice for 401 k contributions, real estate, investing, and financial planning.
- Payroll and payroll taxes.
- Regular meetings to discuss the performance of the practice and to recommend improvements where needed.

During the initial start-up phase of the practice, advisors, such as brokers, real estate agents, and lenders, will be utilized. A local bank can also be a resource for options on establishing a line of credit. Most lenders will require a business plan or pro-forma of the business. This will be discussed later in Chapter 9, Financing the Medical Practice.

Other Advisors to Consider

The following are other advisors to consider to assist the practice:

1. **Insurance Agent or Broker.** There are several types of insurance that must be selected for the new practice. Following are the types of insurance that will need to be considered:

- Malpractice
- General liability and property insurance
- Employee health insurance
- Disability insurance
- Workers compensation insurance
- Life insurance

Choosing an agent or broker can be very critical. There are also a number of considerations to ensure that the practice is properly insured. For example, will the insurance plan cover the cost to recreate medical records if they become destroyed? Is the practice protected if the information system becomes damaged and the practice is unable to recover critical information to be collected for services? Who is responsible if other tenants in the building flood the office space? Who is responsible if a patient falls in the parking lot or just outside the office? Is the practice protected from breaching a patient's privacy as mandated under the Health Insurance Portability and Accountability Act (HIPAA).

2. **Practice Management Consultant.** Many physicians and physician groups go through the entire practice cycle without ever seeking the assistance of an experienced practice management consultant. Unfortunately, these physicians probably spend many hours of their own valuable time and effort on projects that a consultant could handle in a fraction of the time. In particular, a physician new to practice or in a practice transition will benefit greatly by using an experienced consultant. Besides offering operational advice and organizing the practice set up, the seasoned consultant can develop policies and procedure manuals, fee schedules, employee handbooks, and job descriptions for the practice. For established or existing practices, engaging a consulting firm to complete an operational assessment can uncover areas where practice efficiencies can improve and where revenue can be enhanced for improvements in billing and collections procedures.

When selecting the practice consultant, ask candidates for the names of other physicians whom the consultant helped. Talking with these references provides a feel for the consultant's knowledge, the nature of the assignments, and the success of the project in which the physician received assistance.

Use a written agreement (between the physician and the consulting firm) listing, as specifically as possible, what you expect to be achieved. Corresponding to this list, the consulting firm should state exactly the work they will provide, including a time line for completing the work.

Practice management consultants are numerous; thus, check their references carefully. Listed below are a few entities with nationwide services you may wish to contact.

The Coker Group
11660 Alpharetta Highway, Suite 710
Roswell, GA 30076
(800) 345-5829
www.cokergroup.com

AMA KnowledgeLink
515 North State Street
Chicago, IL 60610
(312) 464-5000
www.amasolutions.com/
knowledge/current.shtml

Medical Group Management Association
104 Inverness Terrace East
Englewood, CO 80112-5306
(877) 275-6462
www.mgma.com

CONCLUSION

The more you know about yourself and the better prepared you are to start out in medical practice, the more likely and sooner you will achieve success. By understanding the scope of the start-up and by working through a methodical timetable, you will be able to check off the tasks as you accomplish them and be fully equipped on opening day to see your first patients.

Begin the start-up process by establishing your relationships with trusted advisors and maintain them throughout the years. While professional advisors may appear to be expensive, the knowledge and expertise of a consultant who is experienced in setting up a medical practice will more than offset the cost. In addition, it will save you valuable time and provide the security of knowing the consultant is working from experience and proven techniques gained from years of establishing successful medical practices.

The next chapter will explore the various options that are available for structuring and positioning your practice as a viable entity.

chapter 2

Choosing an Organizational Structure

INTRODUCTION

In starting a medical practice, one of the first questions to ask is "What form of legal entity should be used?" or "How should I organize my business?" Also, as the practice grows and changes, continuously revisit the issue of whether the chosen entity is still the best form of organization for the business.

The purpose of this chapter is to give an overview of various business structures and models that may be chosen when establishing your medical practice. Each has steps to be taken and procedures to follow. They also have advantages and disadvantages to consider that will have long-term effects on the operations. The important point is to be informed so that the right choices can be made to fit your style and personality.

TYPES OF MEDICAL PRACTICES

When considering starting your own practice, carefully consider the sort of entity to ensure the greatest success. Under the existing laws, there are four major types of medical practices that can be established. Following is a brief overview.

- **Sole Proprietorship (one physician).** This type of business has one owner who makes all decisions. Few legal formalities are required. All income or losses, which include deductions for business expenses, belongs to you. Moreover, the sole proprietor is personally liable for all debts, loans, and liabilities.
- **Partnership (group practice).** A general partnership is an association of two or more persons as co-owners who contribute money or property to form a business. The partnership must file an annual tax return (ie, Form 1065), but the business itself is not taxed. Instead, its net income (or loss) is attributed (although not necessarily distributed) directly among the partners in proportion to the investment; individually, they report the profit or loss on their own tax return (ie, Schedule E, Form 1040).
- **Corporation (solo or group practice).** A corporation is a legal entity that is authorized by a state to operate under the rules of

the entity's charter. The most complex business organization, a professional corporation is formed by a group of investors and has the rights and liabilities separate from the individuals involved.

- **Limited Liability Company (group practice).** Shareholders of limited liability corporations are not personally liable for debts of the company.

Group practices can have several variations, including nonprofit practices, foundations, and associations, in addition to the more typical partnerships and corporate practices. Your legal and tax advisors can help determine which structure meets your specific needs. The way in which you structure your practice will depend upon your personality, comfort level, and personal preferences. The following is a basic description of each structure.

Sole Proprietorship

"A sole proprietorship is an unincorporated business that is owned by one individual. Its primary advantage is its ease of formation—it is the simplest form of business organization to start and maintain. The business has no existence apart from you, the owner. Its primary disadvantages are that it can have only one owner. Its liabilities are your personal liabilities, and you undertake the risks of the business for all assets owned, whether used in the business or personally owned. You include the income and expenses of the business on your own tax return."[1]

With autonomy as the major advantage, a solo practice allows the physician to be in control and to establish practice guidelines, office hours, policies, and procedures as preferred. Good candidates for a solo practice tend to be independent and entrepreneurial, and enjoy the business side of operating a practice. This would be a good time to refer back to the self-assessment tool in Chapter 1, Table 1-1, Practice Style Decision-Maker, to see how you scored. You may even want to reconsider some of your answers now that you know more about what is involved.

In a sole proprietorship, the physician is personally liable for all the debt and legal technicalities of the practice. The tax status is simplified in that the physician uses the Internal Revenue Service (IRS) Form 1040, Schedule C (ie, Profit and Loss from Business) to file practice earnings and expenses.

In addition to financial exposure, the disadvantages of solo practice are not having others to share the responsibilities, both for

---

[1] Internal Revenue Service. Sole Proprietorships, Small Business/Self-Employed. *The Digital Daily.* http://www.irs.gov/businesses/display/o,,il=2&genericID=20859,00.html. 07/25/02.

delivering medical care and running an office. This also means that covering the practice during the evening or during vacations will also be your responsibility. It can initially mean less personal time for your family and yourself. As the practice grows, you will likely employ another physician or add mid-level providers to offset the obligations for call coverage and to cover your time off.

Another disadvantage is the potential inability to enter managed care plans.

Figure 2-1 is a chart that specifies the advantages and disadvantages of a sole proprietorship. More pros and cons are covered later in this chapter.

Getting Started
To start a sole proprietorship, simply begin conducting business. Open a separate bank account to keep track of the practice's finances, and keep records of all of the expenses and revenues connected with running the practice.

A sole proprietorship is usually operated under the name of the individual owner, although other names can be used. If the individual owner's name is not used, a *fictitious name* certificate will need to be filed in the town, city, or county where the practice is located. Take care to select a name that is not the same or similar to another practice and avoid using *incorporated* or *company* unless the business is actually a corporation.

Call local government offices for information and application forms that are required in your state and locality (eg, business licenses, zoning occupancy permits, tax registrations, etc).

Control
As owner of all assets of the business, the sole proprietor controls the business. Employees may help manage the practice, but the owner has legal responsibility for the employees' decisions and ultimate control over the business.

FIGURE 2-1

Sole Proprietorship—Advantages and Disadvantages

Advantages	Disadvantages
Control	**Funding**
A sole proprietor controls the money and makes the decisions.	Obtaining capital can be a challenge due to fewer assets.
Easy to set-up	**Threats**
Few legal restrictions. Simple to start and maintain.	If the owner becomes injured or incapacitated, the business will suffer.
Flexibility	**Liability**
The sole proprietor owns the business.	The owner is 100% responsible and takes all the risks.
Easier Taxes	**Responsibilities**
No separate tax form required.	One-hundred percent of the decisions will rest with the owner.

Liability

The sole proprietor has unlimited personal responsibility if the practice fails or has losses and can be sued individually by creditors for non-payment. The business creditors can go against both the business's assets and the owner's personal assets, including bank account, car, or house. Likewise, personal creditors can make claims against the sole proprietor's practice's assets.

Insurance may be purchased to cover many of the risks of a sole proprietorship. However, the owner is personally liable for operating losses.

Continuity and Transferability

As long as its owner is alive and desires to continue the practice, the sole proprietorship can exist. The sole proprietorship ceases to exist when the owner dies. At that point, the assets and liabilities become part of the owner's estate.

All or a portion of the assets of the practice can be freely transferred to another person.

Taxes

All income from the practice is taxed at applicable individual tax rates, with income and allowable business expenses reflected on the individual tax return. No separate federal income tax return is required of the sole proprietor, although the proprietor must pay self-employment tax on the business income.

Pros and Cons

Following are the pros involved with establishing a sole proprietorship:

■ Inexpensive to start
■ Simple to run

The cons of owning a sole proprietorship are as follows:

■ Owner has unlimited personal liability for business
■ Business has unlimited liability for owner's personal liabilities
■ Ownership is limited to one person

Partnership

A partnership is the relationship existing between two or more persons who join to carry on a trade or business. Each person contributes money, property, labor, or skill, and expects to share in the profits and losses of the business. [2] Not a taxable entity, in a partnership, the partners include their share of the income or loss on

---

[2] Internal Revenue Service. Partnerships, Small Business/Self-Employed. *The Digital Daily*. http://www.irs.gov/businesses/display/0,,il=2&genericID=20858,00.html. 07/25/02.

their individual tax returns. Partners are not employees and should not be issued an IRS Form W-2 in lieu of Form 1065, Schedule K-1, for distributions or guaranteed payments from the partnership.

Partners invest in their business to make a profit and are equally responsible for the success or failure of it. It is always a good idea to go into a partnership with someone you can trust and count on to make the same commitments and sacrifices that are needed to have a successful medical practice.

It is advisable to have a written agreement signed by all partners addressing major issues relating to the practice, including:

■ How much time and/or money the partners will contribute to the practice
■ How business decisions will be made
■ How profits and losses will be shared
■ What will happen to the practice and to a partner's share of the business if that partner dies, becomes disabled, or stops working/contributing to the practice
■ How long the partnership will exist
■ When the partnership will make distributions (ie, payments of income earned based upon partnership share) to its partners

Other issues the partnership agreement may address are:

■ Name
■ Types of partners (eg, general, limited, active, silent)
■ Draws and salaries
■ Dispute resolution
■ Arbitration
■ Authority

Partnerships in medical practice can form by two or more established physicians coming together to do business, or when an existing solo practitioner or established practice is seeking to replace retiring members or to grow or expand. One advantage of a partnership is that there is usually a period of employment prior to the "buy in," which would allow the physician time to evaluate the job. Figure 2-2 addresses some of the advantages and disadvantages of a partnership.

Types of Partnerships
Partnerships are either general partnerships or limited partnerships. A *general partnership* is created when two or more individuals agree to create a business and jointly own the assets, profits, and losses. To create a *limited partnership* requires following certain steps set out in each particular state's statues. Partnerships offer the advantage of more than one owner. As a disadvantage, general partners are personally responsible for losses and other obligations of the business.

Figure 2-2

Partnership—Advantages and Disadvantages

Advantages	Disadvantages
👍 **Equal Rights** Each partner has equal rights in management and conduct of partnership.	👎 **Liable for Acts of the Partnership** Each partner is also liable for acts of commission or omission assumed by the partnership as a whole.
👍 **Shared Decision-Making** All partners must give consent when bringing in new partners.	👎 **Liability for Partner's Acts** The partnership can neither sue or be sued per se. However, each partner is liable for any suit against a partner if the suit concerns the principal nature of the business — in this case medicine.
👍 **Shared Rights** Partners have the right to a formal accounting of partnership affairs.	👎 **Equal Benefits** A partner who does not contribute equally to the practice will still expect equal benefits.
👍 **Shared Responsibilities** Each partner has the responsibility to sustain a fiduciary relationship with the other partners.	👎 **Shared Failure** Compensation is based on group performance. If a partner fails to achieve financial success, the group income will suffer.
👍 **Less Risk** Partnership profits must be divided equally among the partners or based on a prearranged schedule.	👎 **Goodwill not portable** Upon leaving a partnership, rarely will the physican recoup an investment, especially the goodwill that may now be associated with the practice as a result of all efforts.
👍 **Responsibilities** Financial responsibilities are shared.	👎 **Exposure to loss** If a partner leaves, the group will be affected as a result of bearing the overhead structure to which the departing physician contributed.

Getting Started

To start a general partnership, agree—orally or in writing—with one or more individuals to jointly own and share the profits of a business.

A limited partnership consists of one or more *general partners* (ie, those who are generally liable for the business) and one or more *limited partners* (ie, those who have limited liability). It must follow the statutory requirements of the state or it will be treated as a general partnership. (See more about limited partnerships and limited corporations later in this chapter.)

Partnerships often use the name of the partners as the name of the business. If all the partners' names are not used, or if none of the partners' names are used, a *fictitious name* certificate may need to be filed.

Many states require partnerships to file certificates either with the local government or in the office of the secretary of state or its equivalent. Check with the local government office to determine the state's requirements.

The partnership should keep separate bank accounts and financial records for the practice so that the partners know of the entity's profits and losses.

Control

The partnership agreement should state what percentage of the practice and profits each partner would own. Otherwise, each partner will own an equal portion of the business and profits and liabilities of the practice.

The agreement should also specify who would control and manage the business of the partnership. Otherwise, all general partners have equal control and management rights and must consent and agree to partnership decisions. Any partner can bind the partnership and the individual partners to contracts or legal obligations, even without the approval of the other partners.

In a limited partnership, the general partners handle the management and control of the business. State law restricts the types of control and management the limited partners can undertake without jeopardizing the limited partnerships' existence.

Liability

A general partnership has characteristics of both a separate legal entity and a group of individuals. The partnership can own property and conduct business as a separate legal entity. The general partners are "jointly and severally liable" for the partnership (ie, all of the partners are liable together and each general partner is individually liable for all of the obligations of the partnership). This means that a creditor of the partnership could require you individually to pay all the money the creditor is owed. Your partners would then reimburse you for their share of the debt or loss.

Before joining a general partnership, determine whether your partners can financially afford to share the losses of the partnership. If you are the only partner with any assets or money, the creditors of the partnership can require you to pay them, and you will be unable to get reimbursement from your partners.

Limited partners do not have personal liability for the business of the partnership. Limited partners are at risk only to the extent of their previously agreed-upon contributions to the partnership.

Continuity and Transferability

A partnership exists as long as the partners agree it will and as long as all of the general partners remain in the partnership. If a general partner departs, the partnership dissolves and the assets of the partnership must be sold or distributed to pay first the creditors and then the partners. The partnership agreement may provide for the continuation of the business by the remaining partners, in which case it may not have to be sold upon the withdrawal of a general partner. The departing general partner is entitled to an accounting to determine shares of the assets and profits of the partnership. The partnership agreement should also cover how partners will be paid for their shares of the partnership upon departure or death.

The partnership agreement should state whether a partner could sell his or her partnership shares. In many states, the sale or transference of a partnership share requires the consent of all the other partners. Even if a partner does transfer a share of the partnership, he or she will remain personally liable for the business losses incurred prior to the sale of that interest.

Taxes

Although a partnership tax return is filed (for informational purposes only), each partner individually pays taxes on his or her share of the practice income. In certain cases, a partner may be required to pay tax on income from the partnership, even without having received any of the income. Partners must also pay self-employment tax on their partnership income.

Pros and Cons

The following are a few of the pros involved with partnerships:

- Very flexible form of business
- Permits ownership by more than one individual
- Avoids double taxation
- Has few legal formalities for its maintenance

The cons of becoming part of a partnership include:

- Partners have unlimited personal liability for business losses
- Partnership is legally responsible for the business acts of each partner
- General partnership interest may not be sold or transferred without consent of all partners
- Partnership dissolves upon death of a general partner

Corporate Practice

The stock corporation has certain advantages that make it worth considering as a business form. A corporation is considered a separate legal entity; the owners of the corporation (eg, shareholders, stockholders) are not personally responsible for the losses of the business. Although usually owned by more than one individual, it is possible for only one individual to create and own 100 percent of a corporation.

A stock corporation may elect Subchapter S status for tax purposes, if it meets the following requirements:

1. Corporation has no more than 35 shareholders
2. Corporation has only one class of stock
3. All shareholders are United States residents, either citizens or resident aliens
4. All shareholders are individuals
5. Corporation operates on a calendar year financial basis

Corporate practice reduces the personal and financial risk to the individual physician, while providing opportunities to shelter income through a qualified retirement program. However, incorporating can be a complicated undertaking because the corporation is considered a distinct legal entity with no ties to any individuals. Figure 2-3 lists the advantages and disadvantages of the corporate practice.

Getting Started

Doing business as a corporate entity calls for compliance with your state's requirements for creating the corporation. Physicians may be required to do business as a professional corporation. The shareholders or stockholders must agree on the following to create a corporation:

■ The name of the business

■ The total number of shares of stock the corporation can sell or issue (ie, *authorized shares*)

■ The number of shares of stock each of the owners will buy

■ The amount of money or other property each owner will contribute to buy his or her shares of stock

■ The business in which the corporation will engage (ie, medical practice)

■ Who will manage the corporation (ie, directors, officers)

Once these issues are settled, shareholders must prepare and file articles of incorporation or a certificate of incorporation with the corporate office of the state. Most states charge an initial fee for

FIGURE 2-3

Corporate Practice—Advantages and Disadvantages

Advantages	Disadvantages
👍 **Protection** There is limited liability to the individual physician.	👎 **Limitations** Only physicians can be shareholders.
👍 **Benefits** The corporation pays benefits (ie, medical insurance, life insurance, disability), making it an expense that is tax deductible.	👎 **Double Taxation** Physician salaries and profits of the corporation are taxed. Assuring that the corporation has small, if any, profit can offset this.
👍 **Centralized Management** Authority and responsibilities are assigned to the appropriate parties, leaving physician to concentrate on patients.	👎 **High Cost** It is quite costly to establish a corporation. Legal fees are high (eg, attorneys' fees are approximately $250 plus per hour) and Social Security payments are higher for the physicians.
👍 **Continuity of Life/Transferable Ownership** The corporation will last beyond the careers of the present physicians. Ownership interest can be transferred easily through the sale of stock representing the value of the corporation's assets.	👎 **Highly Structured** Managing a corporation requires extensive organization (eg, board meetings with accurate minutes, formal notices of annual and quarterly meetings, election of officers, proper revision of bylaws and articles of incorporation, as required). A biannual registration fee of $150 to medical licensing board is required.

filing the corporate documents and an annual fee for allowing the corporation to continue. States vary on rules and fees; to determine what fees will apply, call your state's corporate commission or secretary of state to determine what fees will apply.

The corporation will also need *bylaws*—a set of rules of procedure by which the corporation is run. Bylaws include rules regarding stockholder meetings, director meetings, the number of officers in the corporation, and the responsibilities of each officer.

As a legal entity separate from its owners, the corporation will need a separate bank account and separate records. The money and property that the shareholders pay to buy their stock, and the assets and money that are earned by the corporation, are owned by the corporation and not by the shareholders.

Corporate documents sent to the state must include the name of the corporation. The state will reject the name that is chosen if it is already in use by another company. Most states can tell the caller by telephone if the selected name is available. If possible, avoid using a name that is similar to existing practices.

Control

Shareholders elect, by a majority of the outstanding shares, a group of individuals to act as the board of directors, with ultimate control belonging to those who hold a majority of the shares. Directors' terms of service often are for more than one year and are usually staggered to provide continuity. Shareholders can elect themselves to be on the board of directors. Major decisions must be approved by the shareholders, such as amendments to the articles of incorporation, merger with another practice, and dissolving the corporation. States vary on their requirements for voting, decision-making, and other provisions. Seek professional advice for options that are permissible in your state.

The board of directors makes major decisions of the corporation. Required to meet at least once a year, each director is given one vote; usually the vote of a majority of the directors is sufficient to approve a decision. Directors may be paid, although not required. The board elects the officers of the corporation, usually a president, vice president, secretary, and treasurer. In some states, one person may hold any or all of these offices.

Officers of the corporation are responsible for running the day-to-day business of the corporation. Although they often are employees of the corporation and receive a salary, they can be non-employees and/or serve without pay. The shareholders can be elected as officers.

Stockholder-employees may be paid with wages or a salary for work performed and as a dividend or distribution on the stock.

Dividends must be paid equally, usually as an amount per share. The board of directors makes decisions about payment of dividends. Shareholders have no rights to any of the money of the corporation other than salary or wages if dividends are not distributed. As a separate legal entity, the money it makes belongs to the corporation.

Liability

As a legal entity apart from its owners, creditors of the corporation may look only to the corporation and the business assets for payment. Individual shareholders are not personally liable for the losses of the business if the corporation is properly established and operated. The shareholders' risk is limited to their investment in the corporation, provided that the shareholders comply with the statutory requirements for the corporation, which includes keeping the money, accounts, and assets separate from their personal accounts. However, if the shareholders personally underwrite (ie, guarantee the obligations of the corporation in order to borrow money or to rent space), then they are legally responsible for the obligations they have personally guaranteed. Shareholders' loans to the corporation are subordinated to other loans of the corporation if the business fails.

Continuity and Transferability

Corporate existence lasts as long as its shareholders consider it to serve its purpose. Stockholders can transfer ownership, or corporations can add owners by sale of all or a portion of the stock, either by selling stock directly from the corporation or by having the current owners sell some of their stock. (Before selling shares of stock to outsiders, check to see whether federal or state securities laws permit the sale.)

Medical practices that are corporations are often owned by a small group of shareholders who all work in the practice. Often they formally agree to certain restrictions on the sale of their shares, so that they can control who owns the practice.

Taxes

The corporation must file its own income tax returns and pay taxes on its profits. It must report all income it has received from its business and may deduct certain expenses it has paid in conducting its business.

Dividends paid to shareholders by the corporation are taxed to each shareholder individually, which is in effect a *double taxation*. Both the corporation pays taxes on its profits, and the shareholders must pay taxes on the dividends paid to them from the profits. Taxes are based on personal salary and corporate profits and require separate tax returns.

Generally, a Subchapter S corporation does not pay taxes on the income generated by the business. Income or losses are passed through to the individual shareholders and reported on their tax returns, divided among the shareholders based upon the percentage of stock. Shareholders may be required to pay tax on the income of a Subchapter S corporation even if not paid any dividends or distributions from the corporation.

Pros and Cons
The following are the pros related to forming a corporate practice:

- Provides limited liability to owners
- Is easy to transfer ownership
- Is easy to add additional owners/investors

The cons of establishing a corporate practice include:

- Is more costly to set up and maintain
- Requires separate tax returns
- Is subject to double taxation

OTHER BUSINESS MODELS AND ALTERNATIVES

Sole proprietors can enjoy some of the advantages of a partnership through alternative arrangements. Similar to limited partnerships are limited liability corporations (LLCs); however, some guidance and caution are warranted in these models, as explained in the following section.

Limited Liability Corporation

Although not legal in every state, the IRS has recently approved a fourth option, the limited liability corporation, as an approved corporate structure. It provides the owners with the best advantages of both the corporation and the partnership. Check with your attorney or legal department to verify that your state recognizes the LLC as a legal corporation. While the LLC structure is appropriate for most forms of business, state law in some states set up a parallel structure for doctors, lawyers, accountants, and other professionals called Professional LLC or PLLC.

Under Professional LLC provisions, members are not liable for the overall obligations of the LLC. However, each member is liable for any negligence, wrongful act, or misconduct committed by him or by any person under his direct supervision while rendering services on behalf of the LLC.

Membership in the Professional LLC may only be transferred to other professionals who are eligible. At least one of the professionals forming an LLC must be authorized (licensed) to render professional services in the state where the LLC is formed. In the case of a medical PLLC, all members must be licensed in that state.

The following are the advantages of forming an LLC:

- The personal liability of each member of an LLC is limited to his or her personal investment in the LLC. This means that no member of the LLC is personally liable for the debts of the entire organization.
- The LLC offers pass-through tax benefits (ie, there is no entity-level tax on the entity's income, but only a tax on the individual's share of the entity's income).

Other notable features about an LLC are:

- **Ownership.** Partners and shareholders (members) are owners of an LLC. To ensure pass-through tax benefits, membership in the LLC may not be transferred without consent of a majority of the members of the LLC. Anyone can be an LLC member.
- **Management.** The LLC may be managed by its members or by one or more managers appointed by the members.
- **Rights and Responsibilities.** LLC members generally vote in proportion to their ownership interests, and all matters require the approval of a majority of the members. As with any other type of business, the LLC must obtain a certificate of authority to conduct business in another state. However, the other state must recognize the LLC structure and its qualification requirements.

Getting Started

For information on how to start an LLC, see the *Getting Started* section under *Partnerships* and *Corporations* earlier in this chapter.

Control

For information on the issues of control with regard to an LLC, see the *Control* sections under *Partnerships* and *Corporations* earlier in this chapter.

Liability

For more information on LLC liability issues, see the *Liability* sections under *Partnerships* and *Corporations* earlier in this chapter.

Continuity and Transferability

For more information on Continuity and Transferability of an LLC, see the *Continuity and Transferability* sections under *Partnerships* and *Corporations* earlier in this chapter.

Taxes

An LLC may be a sole proprietorship, a corporation, or a partnership. (A minimum of two members is required for federal tax purposes to operate an LLC as a partnership.) Consequently, the applicable tax forms, estimated tax payment requirements, and related tax publications depend upon whether the LLC operates as a sole proprietorship, corporation, or partnership. The default entity for federal tax treatment of an LLC with two or more members is a partnership. The default entity of an limited liability partnership (LLP) is a partnership and the partnership tax forms, estimated

30

payment requirements, and partnership publications apply. An LLC and/or LLP makes an entity election with Form 8832, Entity Classification Election. [3]

Office-Sharing Arrangements

While this is not a legal structure, some physicians choose to share offices in order to share the cost of operations with another physician. The two parties should maintain a written agreement concerning their arrangement.

Patients should be aware that the two physicians have separate legal entities. If there is no written agreement, and patients assume that the physicians are *partners*, both physicians may be implicated in malpractice litigation. The two parties also need to be mindful of any Stark anti-kickback regulations, such as allowing another physician to share office space, supplies, staff, or other resources in exchange for their referrals. Doing this will be a direct violation of the law. For a complete listing of the Stark Law regulation go to http://oig.hhs.gov/. Again, this just underscores the importance of establishing a written agreement.

The written agreement should include the following:

- A statement of purpose (eg, "This agreement is solely for the purpose of sharing office space for the practice of medicine and is not an agreement creating a partnership between the two parties.")
- Names of the parties involved, the location of the office, whether both parties enter into the lease, or one physician sublets or leases a part of his owned space to another physician; the term of the lease agreement
- How the office space will be allocated
- How expenses will be allocated (ie, equally, based on allocated space, by a predetermined formula, borne separately)
- Allocation of personnel (Sharing staff members carries some risks for the physicians. It is recommended that each physician employ his or her own employees.)
- Provisions for purchase of equipment and furniture
- General liability insurance/health insurance coverage (This may be purchased as one policy at considerable savings to both physicians. Check with your insurance agent.)
- Provisions in case of the death of one of the physicians
- Provisions for one of the physicians ending the agreement (eg, assignment of telephone number, division of furniture and equipment, substitution of another tenant)

---

[3] Internal Revenue Service. Small Business/Self-Employed. *The Digital Daily*. http://www.irs.gov/businesses/display/0..il=2&genericId=20857,00.html. 07/25/02.

TABLE 2-1

Comparison of Legal Entities[4]

	Difficulty and cost to form	Difficulty and cost to maintain	Risk of owner liability	Difficulty of tax preparation	Flexibility of ownership; bringing in new owners	Cost of terminating business
Sole Proprietorship	Low	Low	High	Low	Low	Low
Partnership	Low to Moderate	Low	High	Moderate	Moderate	High
Corporation	High	High	Low	High	High	High
Sub S Corporation	High	High	Low	High	Low	High

COMPARING LEGAL ENTITIES

In summary, Table 2-1, Comparison of Legal Entities, is a table comparing a number of factors of these business models to be considered when setting up your medical practice.

For more information, refer to the Small Business Administration's *Selecting the Legal Structure for Your Business* at http://www.sba.gov/library/pubs/mp-25.pdf. Because state laws vary, consult with an attorney to attain the legal advice necessary for establishing your practice.

CONCLUSION

The best way to make a good decision about choosing the organizational structure for your practice is to have a broad base of knowledge of the advantages and disadvantages of each business entity. Then, an informed decision can be made based upon one's own personality and preferences. Whatever organizational structure you select, you will need to adhere to the tax requirements and comply with the regulations that apply to that legal entity.

---

[4] U.S. Small Business Administration. *Selecting the Legal Structure for Your Business.* http://www.sba.gov/library/pubs/MP-25.PDF. 07/25/02.

Selecting Your Professional Path

INTRODUCTION

Chapter 1, *Getting Started*, and Chapter 2, *Choosing an Organizational Structure*, present the various options for going into practice, weighing the pros and cons of each opportunity. Basically, although the business model of the entity may vary, the three primary options to consider are the following:

- **Option One:** Solo Practice
- **Option Two:** Group Practice (includes partnerships)
- **Option Three:** Employment

CHOOSING A STRUCTURE

With the three aforementioned options in mind, how do you know which is right for you? Since you selected a book titled *Starting a Medical Practice*, the assumption is that most of our readers want to do just that—start their own practice instead of joining an existing one. The majority of physicians who start a medical practice were first employed before going out on their own. Regardless of where you began, if you are going to start your own practice you need to carefully consider which option is right for you. Table 3-1, Practice Option Grid, analyzes the differences in practice opportunities.

Recent Trends in Physician Employment Initiatives

In the early 1990s, according to the American Medical Association's Health Policy Research Center, the proportion of self-employed physicians dropped from 68.1 percent in 1990 to 39.4 percent in 1995. Solo practices were less favored because of the expense of operation, excessive paperwork, increasing rules and regulations, and the daily problems of managing employees. Further, solo physicians felt that they would have difficulty in negotiating favorable managed care contracts. Many Physician Practice Management Companies (PPMCs) or group practices were formed as a result. On paper, these organizations had a lot of promise and offered physicians the opportunity to do what they do best—provide medical care to patients. In theory, the PPMCs or group practices would leverage the economies of scale by centralizing the process and functions for running a practice. They would also leverage their strengths in numbers to allay undesirable managed care plans. Even hospitals

TABLE 3-1

Practice Option Grid

	Positives	Negatives
Solo Practice	■ Independence ■ Clinical autonomy ■ Immediate rewards for efficiency	■ Risk for practice and clinical management ■ Must develop own patient base ■ No financial cushion
Small Group Practice	■ Greater role in governance than in larger group ■ Shared risk and overhead	■ Responsible for colleagues' performance ■ Less independence than solo ■ Shared financial losses
Large Group Practice	■ Overhead costs and financial risk spread among more physicians ■ Clinical synergies ■ Referral opportunities	■ Reduced independence ■ Reduced governance role ■ Liability for group financial and clinical performance
Employee Status	■ Low financial risk ■ Guaranteed paychecks ■ Relief from practice administration	■ Limited income growth potential ■ Little independence or control ■ Future tied to organization's success

were buying physician practices and employing physicians to establish provider networks to keep from loosing market share to managed care or competing hospitals. In some cases the hospital would form a Management Service Organization (MSO) that would provide centralized management services.

In the end, with a few exceptions, most of these organizations were not extremely successful. Several issues contributed to their mediocre performance or failure; however, in most cases there were three primary reasons:

1. Mismanagement and excessive overhead.
2. Physicians were paid a salary with no incentives to see patients.
3. Participating in managed care did not give any competitive edge because exclusives were rarely given.

These initiatives also created competition among physicians to contend for managed care contracts. However, in the end everyone agreed to discount fees to participate in the same plan, giving no competitive edge for agreeing to accept less money. Moreover, the practices became consumed and overwhelmed with the guidelines of managed care. In most cases, practices had to add extra employees to do the extra work. As economic pressures mounted and patient care suffered as a result of cutting cost, physicians in the late 1990s began to reconsider their decision to join a group practice or PPMC. Again, while joining a group or a PPMC is still a viable option, it is primarily a starting place for many physicians who eventually start their own practice.

As stated previously, the predominant reason a physician chooses solo practice is to have autonomy—the freedom to establish the practice guidelines, office hours, policies and procedures, and so forth that he or she prefers. Younger physicians seek settings where they can focus on patient care. Solo practice permits the flexibility and personal attention to patients that group practices often forfeit. As a result, an increasing number of physicians are now going back into private practice or repurchasing their practices.

Nonetheless, joining a group practice is still very common for physicians who are just starting their careers. The younger generation of physicians is more likely to compartmentalize their professional and personal lives than are older physicians. They expect to have time for their families and outside interests. Some younger doctors prefer the stability of a group setting to the risks of a solo or partnership setting. Working with technology is comfortable for younger professionals; they are less comfortable with handling paper charts than they are computerized records. On that premise, several points should be contemplated before making the decision to join a group.

The purpose of this chapter is to provide information that will allow you to make an informed decision about joining a group practice. Topics included are the advantages and disadvantages of joining a group (also see Chapter 2, *Choosing an Organizational Structure*), what to look for in a contract, and how to evaluate the character and effectiveness of a group. This chapter will also help you investigate employment opportunities with hospitals and Health Maintenance Organizations (HMOs), and incorporates tips on what to look for in an employment contract.

Group Practice—To Join or Not to Join?

Below are some advantages and disadvantages that are typical for joining a group practice.

Advantages of group practice:

- Fewer problems establishing office operations and building a patient load
- Less initial financing needed
- Less financial risk involved, providing greater initial security
- Regular work schedules, yielding more time for family and personal pursuits
- Shared call coverage for nights, weekends, and holidays
- Coverage for vacations, sick days, and continuing education
- Professional atmosphere and shared knowledge afforded by group relationships
- Greater access to technology and trained personnel
- Increased opportunities to pursue research and/or administrative interests
- Fewer problems involved in retirement or decreased workload
- Greater competitive advantages because of a larger market share

Disadvantages of group practice:

- Loss of autonomy; decisions made by consensus
- Greater potential for conflicts with associates over personal differences, income distribution, group expenditures and investments, group procedures, and policies and philosophies on patient care
- Pressure to refer patients to physicians within the group (especially in a multispecialty group)
- Greater likelihood of impersonality in dealing with patients
- Possible liability for any errors made by associates of losses incurred by the group
- Greater difficulty in effecting change
- Uneven distribution of cases

Finding Information and Opportunities in Group Practice

The following are resources that can be used for finding information and opportunities in a group practice.

- Residency programs
- Medical schools
- Specialty society placement service
- State, county, and local medical societies
- Physician recruiting firms
- Classified ads in journals and metropolitan newspapers
- Hospital administrators or hospital marketing departments
- Chiefs of staff
- Multisite clinic and hospital management firms
- Preferred Provider Organizations (PPOs)
- Health Maintenance Organizations (HMOs)(all types)
- Personal contacts, including pharmaceutical representatives and durable medical equipment representatives
- Established group practices
- American Group Practice Association, Placement Services
- Practice brokers
- Management consultants
- On-line services
- Group Practice Associations

EMPLOYMENT CONTRACT

Understandably, almost every employment contract is written to favor the employer. You must protect your rights, nevertheless, by ensuring that the contract is fairly written.

Before signing any type of employment agreement, know what to look for and how to interpret the contract language. It is also important to understand that you have some room for negotiation. After reading the contract, define any points that cause concern. Rank these concerns in order of importance. Negotiate firmly on the most important issues and be willing to concede in areas of less interest.

Employment contracts generally include the following clauses:

1. The Term of the Contract
   - Does the contract become effective on the date it is signed or on the day you start to work?
   - What is the length of the contract?
   - Does it have an automatic renewal? Is it subject to renegotiation at the time of renewal?

2. Duties
   - What hours is the employee expected to work and what specific call duties will the employee be expected to handle?
   - Is the employee restricted in any way from seeking additional employment outside of the practice?
   - What kinds of patients will be assigned to the employed physician?
   - What restrictions does the physician employee have regarding the acceptance of patients and modes of treatment?
   - What penalties, if any, are incurred if the employee voluntarily terminates employment before the contract expires?
   - What provisions will apply if the employee is called to jury duty? To military duty?

3. Compensation
   - What salary will the employee receive?
   - How will the salary be computed?
   - At what intervals and increments will the salary increase?
   - What incentive bonuses apply and how are they calculated?

4. Benefits
   - Are pension and profit sharing plans available? What is the vesting schedule?
   - Will the employer pay the employee's malpractice insurance premiums?
   - Who pays for *tail* insurance? (See Chapter 8, *Identifying Insurance Requirements*, for discussion of *tail insurance*.)
   - Will the physician employees participate in the group life insurance plan?
   - What additional fringe benefits will the employee receive?
     - Vacation
     - Sick leave/discretionary days
     - CME/conventions/postgraduate work
     - Professional books and periodicals
     - Professional dues
     - Medical equipment

- Office space
- Clerical help
- Automobile allowance
- Moving allowance

5. Buy-In Agreement
   - On what date will the employee be allowed to acquire part ownership in the practice? What percentage of the practice will the employee be able to purchase at buy-in?
   - What will part ownership in the practice entail? Specifically, what percentage of the following will the new partner own?
     - Accounts receivable
     - Equipment
     - Goodwill
     - Supply inventory and prepaid items
     - Office buildings and real estate location
     - Liabilities
   - What will be the cost to the employee to buy into the practice?
   - How will the value of the practice be determined?
   - What are the exact terms of payment of the buy-in?
     - Lump payments or extended payments
     - Rate of interest

6. Covenant Not to Compete (Restrictive Covenant)
   - Will the employee be asked to sign a covenant not to compete? What are the specific terms of such a covenant?
   - How enforceable is a covenant not to compete in the state where signed?
   - Is there a time limit beyond which a signed covenant not to compete no longer applies?
   - Are there any other clauses in this contract that impose certain obligations or restrictions on the employee?
   - Will the employed physician be allowed a trial period before agreeing to a restrictive covenant?
   - Can you buy out of your non-compete clause?

7. Termination
   - Can either the physician or employer terminate the contract with 30 days notice?
   - Does the contract terminate on death of the employee, or will the employee's family or estate be subject to contractual obligations?
   - Upon termination, can the employer hold you accountable for under-performance losses?
   - Under which, if any, of the following conditions will the contract automatically terminate?
     - Loss of hospital privileges

- Suspension, revocation, or cancellation of employee's right to practice medicine
- Employee refuses to follow practice polices or procedures
- Employee commits an act of gross negligence
- Employee is convicted of a crime
- Employee becomes impaired due to alcohol or drug abuse
- Breach of contract terms
- Employee becomes disabled (eg, How many days, etc?)

Understanding Restrictive Covenants

A restrictive covenant, or a covenant not to compete, may be described as an express provision of an employment contract or a partnership agreement that restricts the right of the employee or associate, after the conclusion of his or her term of employment, to engage in a business similar to or competitive with that of the employer, partner, or seller of the practice.

Such restrictions, usually, are limited to a specified time and geographical area. In jurisdictions where there are no statutory limitations on restrictive covenants, the general rule is that the courts will enforce such covenants if they are reasonable in view of all of the circumstances of a particular case. In assessing the reasonableness of a particular restrictive covenant, a court will consider three major tests of reasonableness, as follows:

- It is no greater than necessary to protect the employer in some legitimate interest
- It is not unduly harsh and oppressive on the employee
- It is not injurious to the public interest

Each case is decided individually; differing time limits and geographical restrictions could be judged as reasonable in a particular case. Courts tend to enforce restrictive covenants in contracts more often for the sale of a practice or business than in employment or partnership contracts.

A physician contemplating employment should not sign a contract containing a restrictive covenant without obtaining legal advice. If the employer insists on a covenant, the physician may wish to negotiate the following:

- A trial period before the restrictive covenant becomes operative
- An eventual limitation after which the covenant is no longer in force
- A provision that states that the restrictive covenant is null and void if the employee is discharged without adequate reason, or if the employee leaves for just cause

Income Distribution and Expense Allocation

Some groups pay each physician a salary and a portion of net revenue, if any, that remains after paying expenses and physician salaries. This excess may be paid to each physician equally or distributed according to a formula. If you will be receiving a base salary and participating in the distribution of net revenue, be sure you understand how it is calculated.

Income Distribution

Following are various examples of income distribution that you may encounter in practice options:

- **Equal Distribution.** Each member receives an equal share of the practice revenue.
- **Productivity.** Members are compensated based on the amount they generate in individual patient charges.
- **Formulas.** Several factors, weighed by importance, are used to determine remuneration. Some of these factors are as follows:
  - Goodwill/longevity
  - Stock ownership
  - Productivity
  - Board certification
  - Administrative roles (eg, managing partner, etc)
  - New patients
  - Referral sources
  - Teaching/faculty position

Each factor in the formula is given percentage points. Physicians in the group must decide how many points will be given to each factor. If points are allocated for longevity, there should be a maximum that each doctor can earn.

Note: The Stark II legislation now prevents groups from compensating a physician based on how much revenue that physician generates for ancillary services, such as lab and x-ray. However, revenue from ancillary services may be distributed equally to each physician in the group, regardless of whether he or she generated this revenue.

Methods of Expense Allocation

The following are four methods used to allocate expenses:

- **Equal Assessments.** This is the easiest method. The expenses are subtracted from the gross revenue, and the net income is available for physician distribution.
- **Direct Costs.** Any costs incurred for the benefit of a physician are charged directly to that physician. This allows each physician to have any equipment or personnel that he or she prefers.
- **Indirect Costs.** Costs such as rent, utilities, and maintenance are charged to each physician, usually as a per-square-foot charge. This way, each physician pays only for what he or she uses.

■ **Expenses as a Percentage of Productivity**. Each physician is charged for expenses at the same rate he or she generates income for the group. If the physician generates 40 percent of the income, he or she is charged 40 percent of the expense. In a multispecialty group, the surgical specialists may object to this type of allocation because primary care physicians typically use much more space than other physicians.

Compensation

The following are types of physician compensation:

■ **Guarantees.** Compensation for fundamental work requirements also referred to as base pay. This is generally agreed upon at the time of employment and is regenerated annually.

■ **Productivity Incentives.** Allow for additional compensation for exceeding certain goals. These goals may include cost containment, utilization, patient satisfaction, or revenue.

■ **Benefits.** Your benefit package will come at a cost for any employer and therefore is often considered part of the total compensation. In some cases, benefits can compensate for lost ground by agreeing to less base pay.

You should always know the salary benchmarks for your specialty and market. Practice associations keep updated lists of these benchmarks that you should review before agreeing to your compensation. Conversely, it is important to note that these benchmarks also include statistics on productivity that must be met to achieve the salary benchmarks. In the beginning your patient volume will be less, which you must bear in mind before making any demands to be paid at these benchmark levels.

GROUP PRACTICE QUESTIONNAIRE

Use the questionnaire in Figure 3-1 to gather information about each practice you consider. By accumulating the same information on each, a fair comparison using the same criteria can be generated.

F I G U R E 3-1

Group Practice Questionnaire

General Information

Date: _____

Name of group: _____

Office address: _____

Telephone: _____

Addresses of satellite offices: _____

Name of person to contact for future information: _____

Home telephone number: _____

F IGURE 3-1 *Continued*

Group Structure

What is the legal structure of the group?

❏ Partnership

❏ Professional Corporation

❏ Limited Liability Corporation

❏ Individuals sharing space

Single or multi-specialty? _____

Who are the group's partners and/or principal stockholders?

Name: _____ *Age:* _____ *Gender:* _____ *Specialty:* _____

Name: _____ *Age:* _____ *Gender:* _____ *Specialty:* _____

Name: _____ *Age:* _____ *Gender:* _____ *Specialty:* _____

Who are the employed physicians?

Name: _____ *Age:* _____ *Gender:* _____ *Specialty:* _____

Name: _____ *Age:* _____ *Gender:* _____ *Specialty:* _____

Name: _____ *Age:* _____ *Gender:* _____ *Specialty:* _____

Are there physicians planning to retire? If so, what is the expected date(s) of retirement? _____

_____

Are there plans to increase the size of the group? _____

_____

What is the ultimate goal regarding size? _____

What makes up the group's geographic market area (eg, counties, miles)? _____

_____

What is the population of the group's market area? _____

How many physicians in my specialty, not associated with this group's market area? _____

_____

Area Hospitals

List hospitals where group members have staff privileges.

Name: _____ *# of beds:* _____

Name: _____ *# of beds:* _____

Are there other hospitals in the area? _____

Does the group place restriction on having privileges at other hospitals? _____

Buy-In Opportunities

Does the group offer partnership to all physician employees? _____

What are the criteria for partnership? _____

What are the number of years of employment required? _____

Is buy-in required? _____

Are the buy-in requirements written into the original employment contract? _____

F IGURE 3-1 *Continued*

Practice Styles

What is the ethical orientation of the group (ie, abortions, birth control, euthanasia)? _____

_____

Is there a feeling of compatibility and cooperation among group physicians? _____

Are all group members Board Certified? _____

Do any group members have a particular skill or certification that sets them apart from other specialists in the same field? If so, what are these skills? _____

_____

Are academic appointments encouraged? _____

Are there constraints placed on time spent in teaching activities? _____

Do any of the physicians have personal or practice problems or limitations of which associates should be aware? _____

_____

How many physicians have left the group in the last three years? _____

Were they employees or partner physicians? _____

What were their reasons for leaving? _____

Will the other physicians in the group be introduced before making a decision? _____

Social Interactions

Do the physicians seem to have a good relationship with each other? _____

Is socializing expected or discouraged among physicians? _____

Do spouses socialize with each other? _____

Have the spouses of the group's physicians been introduced? _____

How does the physician's spouse feel about the other spouses that have been introduced? _____

_____

Do any of the physicians have personal/social problems? _____

_____

Income Distribution

How is practice income distributed?

    ❑ *Equally*

    ❑ *Based on productivity*

    ❑ *Based on formula. If formula, what factors are used to determine income?* _____

_____

What method is used to allocate expenses?

    ❑ *Income and expenses shared equally*

    ❑ *Income and expenses based on productivity*

    ❑ *Income based on productivity, expenses shared equally*

        (Read Income Distribution, above, to interpret the answers to these questions.)

F I G U R E 3-1 *Continued*

Office Facilities

What was the first impression of the office appearance? _____

_____

How long has the group practiced at this address? _____

How many square feet are there in the facility? _____

What ancillary services are provided in office? _____ ❏ *X-ray?* ❏ *Laboratory?*

How accessible is the practice location to patients? _____

Are parking facilities adequate? If not, what plans exist to improve this? _____

Will a personal consulting office be available? _____

How many exam rooms does each physicians have? _____

If there are satellite locations, are the physicians rotated through each location? _____

What is the rotation schedule? _____

Is the office clean? _____ *Well organized?* _____ *Well equipped?* _____

Are there plans for future expansion? _____

Is the size of the reception area adequate? _____

Is there adequate seating in the exam rooms (eg, three seats per exam room is average)? _____

_____

Is special equipment available if specialty requires? _____

Is the facility owned by the group, by the physicians personally, or leased from another entity? _____

What is the distance to hospital(s)? _____

Is the practice in a high growth area or in a declining neighborhood? _____

What days and hours are the offices open? _____

Group Governance

How are decisions made within the group?

  ❏ *Majority vote?*

  ❏ *Governing board?*

  ❏ *Senior physicians?*

  ❏ *Informal clique?*

Who makes day-to-day decisions versus long-term decisions or changes? _____

Is there an office manager/administrator? _____

To whom does this person report? _____

Are there regular business meetings? _____

How often are they held? _____

Are all physicians required to attend? _____

Office Personnel

How many employees in the practice? _____ *Clinical* _____ *Administrative* _____

F IGURE 3-1 *Continued*

What is the staff-to-physician ratio? _____

Are physician extenders used? _____ *How many P.A.s ?* _____ *Nurse Practitioners?* _____

Does each physician have a personal clinical assistant? _____

Does the office appear over- or understaffed? _____

How are patients treated by the staff? _____

Does the staff seem efficient, courteous, and professional? _____

How many staff members have left voluntarily within the last year? _____

What were the reasons they left (ask staff members)? _____

_____

_____

How many staff members have been terminated? _____

Have they been replaced? _____

Is there good communication between staff and physicians? _____

Financial Overview

What were the total charges last year? _____

What were the adjusted charges last year (eg, after contractual write-offs, such as Medicare and managed care)? _____

_____

What were the total collections, same period? _____

What were the total expenses? _____

What percent of the total expenses went to rent/mortgage expense? _____

What are the total accounts receivable? _____

What are the total dollars of A/R over 90 days? _____ *Percent of total A/R?* _____

Does the practice have an operational budget? _____

How does it compare with actual figures? _____

Does the group review financials together every month? _____

What reports will be routinely provided? _____

What is the fee schedule? _____

Do all physicians use the same fee schedule? _____

Are billing and collections done in-house? _____

If not, how is it handled? _____

Is the practice computerized? _____

What software is used for practice management? _____

Who handles the payables (eg, office manager, accountant, other)? _____

Who signs the checks? _____

Managed Care/Medicare Participation

Are all physicians participating in Medicare? _____

FIGURE 3-1 *Continued*

What percentage of practice is Medicare? _____

How many managed care contracts does the group have? _____

What percentage of total patients are on managed care plans? _____

How many plans have at least 20% of the group's patient base? _____

Does any MCO have more than 20% of the group's patient base? _____

Which ones? _____

Does the group have any capitated contracts? _____

How is information about each managed care contract tracked? _____

Does becoming a part of this group make one eligible to see patients on these contracts immediately? _____

Patient Distribution

How are new patients distributed if no preference is given? _____

How is the patient load distributed? _____

How are managed care patients distributed in a group contract? _____

In a single specialty group, how are the unusual cases distributed? _____

Who sees nursing home patients? _____

What is the current call schedule rotation? _____

Malpractice Issues

What has been the group's malpractice experience? _____

Are any malpractice suits pending? _____

Are any considered to have merit? _____

Are any liabilities retroactive? _____

CONCLUSION

If starting your medical practice means joining a group or affiliating with an existing organization, you will need to know a great deal about employment agreements and compensation arrangements. Gather all the facts and assess the conditions of employment before signing on with an existing practice to make sure that the organization is a good fit for your practice style and goals.

chapter 4

Regulations and Licensing Requirements

INTRODUCTION

One of the first challenges of starting a medical practice is learning the scores of rules and regulations that govern health care. Health care is one of the most highly regulated industries in the nation, with many exposures to liabilities and bureaucracies involved. Further, rules are constantly changing which requires continuous education for the practitioner and practice staff. However, with the proper resources, you can easily maneuver your way through the minefield with few wounds.

These laws reside at all levels, which include local, state, and federal procedures. To have one source available with the requirements of every regulation would require a huge volume, with information of immeasurable proportions. The purpose of this chapter, therefore, is to provide a resource directory for regulations required for starting a practice and beyond. Bear in mind that in some cases the regulation may not be entirely applicable. For example, Joint Commission on Accreditation of Healthcare Organizations (JCAHO) regulations apply only if your practice is owned by a JCAHO-approved hospital. In any case, we want to provide you with a comprehensive listing of necessary resources for these regulations for starting your practice and ongoing compliance.

Regulations can be overwhelming. Our advice is to become familiar with the basics, know where to find additional answers when you need them, and, if in doubt, go find out from the proper resource.

REGULATIONS FOR STARTING A MEDICAL PRACTICE

The resource and information that follows are requirements for setting up a medical practice, followed by resources for ongoing regulations.

Employer Identification Number (EIN)

As an employer, you will need an Employer Identification Number (EIN). All correspondence with the IRS and all tax payments must reference this EIN. To apply for an EIN, fill out Form SS-4, which may be obtained at any IRS or Social Security Administration Office. The telephone number and address for the local IRS Service Center can be found in the telephone book under state and/or federal government listings (blue pages). Once the application form has been completed and mailed, it takes approximately five weeks to receive the EIN.

The EIN can also be applied for by telephone. All telephone applicants immediately receive their EIN. Complete the Form SS-4 before calling the IRS Service Center for your state. When the EIN is obtained by telephone, the completed form must be mailed or faxed within 24 hours.

When applying for an EIN, the IRS will send you a payment coupon book (Form 8109) that is to be used for depositing withholding taxes.

The following is the EIN contact information:

Internal Revenue Service (Treasury Dept.)
1111 Constitution Ave., NW
Washington, DC 20224
(800) 823-1040
http://www.ustreas.gov

State Tax Identification Number

A State Tax Number may also be needed. Check with your accountant to be certain that all required identifying numbers for establishing a medical practice in your state have been received.

State Medical License

Call the State Board of Medical Examiners to obtain the necessary forms and a list of any backup documents that may be needed to apply for your state license. For a complete Internet listing of contact information for the Board of Medical Examiners in your state, go to Resources at http://www.cokergroup.com or the Federation of State Medical Boards at http://www.fsmb.org.

Medical Staff Privileges

Before hospital medical staff privileges are awarded, you must be licensed to practice medicine in your state. Visit each hospital in the area where you need to obtain staff privileges. Complete the necessary credentialing forms and collect any other documents that may be needed for attaining admitting privileges. If you are joining a group practice and need to be on call, temporary privileges may be awarded until a license is received.

Federal Narcotics License/Drug Enforcement Administration Number

Under the Controlled Substances Act of 1970, if you have never had a Drug Enforcement Administration (DEA) number, you will need to contact the Department of Justice at the following address to obtain a license to dispense narcotics. New applicants will use DEA Form 224, Application for Registration. This form is for the retail pharmacy, hospital/clinic, practitioner, teaching institution, or mid-level practitioner categories only. The current fee is $210 for three years.

United States Department of Justice
Drug Enforcement Administration
Central Station
P.O. Box 28083
Washington, DC 20038-8083
(202) 307-7725
(800) 882-9539
http://www.deadivision.usdoj.gov/drugreg/index.htm
or
http://www.deadiversion.usdoj.gov/drugreg/reg_apps/index.html

All registrants must report any changes of professional or business address to the DEA. Notification of address changes must be made in writing to the DEA office that has jurisdiction for your registered location. For a list of DEA offices, go to Resources at http://www.cokergroup.com or to the DEA website noted above. Direct requests for the following actions to the address that is listed for your state:

■ Request a modification to your DEA Registration (address change)
■ Request order form books
■ Status of pending application

DEA Form 224A, Renewal Application for Retail Pharmacy, Hospital/Clinic, Practitioner, Teaching Institution, or Mid-Level Practitioner, is coming soon.

State Narcotics License

Some states will also require you to have a state-issued narcotics license. Check to see if the state where you will be practicing requires a state DEA license in addition to the federal license.

Universal Provider Identification Number (UPIN)

The Centers for Medicare/Medicaid Services (CMS), formerly Health Care Financing Administration (HCFA), assigns every physician a Universal Provider Identification Number (UPIN). The number you will be assigned will be your provider number for as long as you are a practicing physician, regardless of where you practice. CMS will assign this number when you apply for a Medicare Provider number. No extra forms are required.

Write to the CMS and request any information available for a new physician.

Centers for Medicare/Medicaid Services
P.O. Box 26676
Baltimore, MD 21207
(410) 786-3000
www.hcfa.gov/medicare/enrollment.html
or
www.cpg.mcw.edu/www/upin.html

CMS regional offices, identified for every state, can be found in the telephone directory in the blue pages under *Government Listings* or on the Internet at http://www.hcfa.gov/regions/roinfo.htm. This information is also available under Resources at www.cokergroup.com.

Medicare Provider Number

If you are starting your own practice and you will be providing medical services to Medicare recipients, you will need to apply for a provider number. The Medicare program has two parts: Part A covers hospital services, and Part B covers physician services. If you already have a Medicare provider number and you are moving to another state, you will be assigned a new provider number for that state.

You will need your state medical license to obtain your Medicare provider number. To apply for the Medicare provider number, contact:

Centers for Medicare/Medicaid Services
P.O. Box 26676
Baltimore, MD 21207
(410) 786-3000
www.hcfa.gov/medicare/enrollment.html
or
www.cpg.mcs.edu/www/upin.html

For questions you may have about who is the Part B carrier (ie, payer and administrator) in your area, contact CMS by telephone or visit their website at the above-provided address.

Medicaid Provider Number

If you will be treating recipients of Medicaid services, you will also need a Medicaid Provider number. It can be obtained from CMS when applying for a Medicare number.

If you are joining a group practice or becoming an employee of a hospital, the Medicare and Medicaid numbers will be linked with a group number for that group or employer. Your employer will help you obtain this provider number. To apply for the Medicaid provider number, contact:

Centers for Medicare/Medicaid Services
P.O. Box 26676
Baltimore, MD 21207
(410) 786-3000
www.cpg.mcs/www/upin.html
or
www.cpg.mcw.edu/www/upin.html

Retired Railroad Employees' Coverage

Travelers Insurance Company covers all retired railroad employees regardless of where they live. Once Travelers assigns a provider number, it remains the same anywhere you practice. The website below has a listing of all the Retired Railroad Board locations in the US:

http://www.rrb.gov/field/html

Business License

Before you open your office you will need a business license, which will be either a city license or a county license, depending on where the practice is located. If the practice is within the city limits, go to the city hall to purchase your license. If the practice is outside the city limits, most likely the license will be obtained by applying at the county courthouse. In rare instances, both a city and a county license may be needed. The cost of the license varies by city and state, but will likely range between $100 and $300. A business license must be renewed every year.

Laboratory License

In October 1988, the federal government passed the Clinical Laboratories Improvement Act (CLIA), which became effective in September 1992. This act requires all physicians' office laboratories to be licensed according to the complexity of the tests they perform. If you are a solo practitioner and plan to do *any* laboratory testing on site, a CLIA number will be needed. Contact CLIA through CMS in your state or on the Internet at: www.hcfa.gov/medicaid/clia/cliahome.htm.

If joining a group, ask what CLIA license the group holds. Table 4-1 contains a list of the different levels of office laboratories and the test each category includes. Determine what tests you will be performing in the office, and apply for the appropriate level of license. Costs are involved in having an in-office laboratory. Each level has a registration fee and an annual inspection fee. Other costs are in proportion to the level of the laboratory and the annual test volume.

Table 4-2 is a tool for assigning CLIA lab compliance.

TABLE 4-1

CLIA Test Categories

Waived	Physician-Performed Microscopy (PPM)
Dipstick/Tablet Urinalysis	Wet Mounts
Ovulation Test Kits	KOH Preps
Urine Pregnancy Tests	Pinworm Preps
Sed Rates (manual)	Fern Tests
Fecal Occult Blood	Post-Coital Qualitative Exam
Glucose Meters	Urine Sediment Exam
Manual Hematocrit	
Hemoglobin ($CuSo_4$)	
Streptococcus Group	
Helicobacter pylori	
Total Cholesterol	
HDL Cholesterol	
Triglycerides	
Glucose	

Moderately Complex	Highly Complex
Most Hematology Instruments	Manual Cell Counts
Manual Diff/Limited ID	Manual Diff/Complete ID
Most Chemistry Tests	Some Esoteric Chemistry Tests
Urine Culture/Colony Count Only	Urine Culture/Organism Identification
Gram Stain/Urethral, Cervical for GC	Gram Stain/Any Other Source
Throat Screen/Hema, Bacitracin, SSA	Throat Culture
GC Screen/Gram Stain, Oxidase	GC Culture/Organism Identification
Rapid Kits/Mono, Strep, Chlamydia	Antibiotic Susceptibility Testing

TABLE 4-2

In-house Lab Compliance Checklist

1. Type of laboratory   Certification number   Current

		Yes	No	N/A
❐ PPMC	_____	❐	❐	❐
❐ Waived	_____	❐	❐	❐
❐ Moderate complexity	_____	❐	❐	❐
❐ High complexity	_____	❐	❐	❐

2. List all waived tests performed (kits):   CPT code used

_____   _____
_____   _____
_____   _____
_____   _____
_____   _____
_____   _____
_____   _____
_____   _____
_____   _____
_____   _____
_____   _____

TABLE 4-2 *Continued*

3. List all PPM performed: CPT code used

    _____   _____

    _____   _____

    _____   _____

    _____   _____

    _____   _____

4. List all other tests performed: CPT code used

    _____   _____

    _____   _____

    _____   _____

    _____   _____

    _____   _____

    _____   _____

    _____   _____

    _____   _____

    _____   _____

5. Name of laboratory director _____

6. Date of last HHS inspection _____
    Results:

    _____

7. Name of testing program _____

8. How many locations owned by this practice? Have a lab? _____

9. Separate license for each?   ❐ Yes   ❐ No

10. Is *pass-through* billing performed?   ❐ Yes   ❐ No

11. How are laboratory fees established? Explain:

    _____

    _____

    _____

12. Are laboratory tests performed credited to the productivity of the physician that ordered the test? Explain:

    _____

    _____

    _____

GENERAL REGULATORY ISSUES AND AGENCIES

The physician must be cognizant of ongoing issues and policies of agencies that regulate the practice of medicine. Particular attention must be paid to decisions and actions by the Center for Medicare and Medicaid Services (CMS); rulings on the Health Insurance Portability and Accountability Act of 1996 (HIPAA); accreditation standards of the Joint Commission on Accreditation of Healthcare Organizations (JCAHO); and activities of the Office of the Inspector General (OIG) and the Department of Justice (DOJ). As an employer, other important agencies to the medical practice are the Occupational Safety and Health Administration (OSHA), the Department of Labor (DOL), and the Equal Employment Opportunity Commission (EEOC). Each of these initiatives is described on the next page.

Center for Medicare and Medicaid Services (CMS)

Previously known as the Health Care Financing Administration (HCFA), the Center for Medicare and Medicaid Services (CMS) provides health insurance through Medicare, Medicaid, and the State Child Health Insurance Program (SCHIP). CMS also performs several quality-focused activities, including regulation of laboratory testing (ie, through CLIA); development of coverage policies; maintains oversight of the survey and certification of nursing homes and continuing care providers; and makes available to beneficiaries, providers, researchers, and state surveyors information about these activities and nursing home quality. For more information, visit www.hcfa.gov.

Health Insurance Portability and Accountability Act (HIPAA)

The Health Insurance Portability and Accountability Act of 1996 (HIPAA) has different meanings to different people. Its purpose is: to improve portability and continuity of health insurance coverage in the group and individual markets; to combat waste, fraud, and abuse in health insurance and health care delivery; to promote the use of medical savings accounts; to improve access to long-term care services and coverage; to simplify the administration of health insurance; and for other purposes. More recently, HIPAA has come to represent privacy initiatives that physicians in medical practice must meet on behalf of their patients. In some way, the entire health care industry is affected by HIPAA in how a patient's health information is transmitted or maintained. Extensive information on HIPAA's impact on the medical practice is available on the Internet at http://www.hcfa.gov/hipaa/hipaahm.htm.

Joint Commission on Accreditation of Healthcare Organizations (JCAHO)

The Joint Commission on Accreditation of Healthcare Organizations (JCAHO) evaluates and accredits nearly 18,000 health care organizations and programs in the United States. JCAHO is an independent, not-for-profit organization, and is the nation's predominant standard-setting and accrediting body in health care. Its mission is to continuously improve the safety and quality of care that is provided to the public through the provision of health care accreditation and related services that support performance improvement in health care organizations. For more information on JCAHO and its effect on the medical practice, visit http://jcaho.org.

Office of Inspector General (OIG)

The Office of Inspector General (OIG) protects the integrity of the Department of Health and Human Services (HHS) programs, as well as the health and welfare of the beneficiaries of those programs. The OIG's responsibility is to report to the Secretary of the

Department and Congress all program and management problems and to offer recommendations to correct them. The OIG's duties are carried out through a nationwide network of audits, investigations, inspections, and other mission-related functions performed by the OIG components. For more information on activities of the OIG and its effect on the medical practice, visit http://oig.hhs.gov.

Department of Justice (DOJ)

The Department of Justice (DOJ) enforces the law and defends the interests of the United States according to the law by providing federal leadership in preventing and controlling crime, seeking just punishment for those who are guilty of unlawful behavior, and ensuring fair and impartial administration of justice for all Americans. For more information, visit http://www/usdoj.gov. The DOJ works with HHS to prevent Medicare fraud and abuse and to bring charges against those who would violate the Medicare and Medicaid programs.

Occupational Safety and Health Administration (OSHA)

The Occupational Safety and Health Administration's (OSHA) mission is to save lives, prevent injuries, and protect the health of America's workers. OSHA and its state partners have approximately 2,100 inspectors, plus complaint discrimination investigators, engineers, physicians, educators, standards writers, and other technical and support personnel spread over more than 200 offices throughout the country. This staff establishes protective standards, enforces those standards, and reaches out to employers and employees through technical assistance and consultation programs. Medical practices are subject to OSHA Guidelines for Bloodborne Pathogens and adherence to OSHA's Hazard Communication Standard. For more information, visit www.osha.gov.

Department of Labor (DOL)

The US Department of Labor fosters and promotes the welfare of the job seekers, wage earners, and retirees of the United States by improving their working conditions, advancing their opportunities for profitable employment, protecting their retirement and health care benefits, helping employers find workers, strengthening free collective bargaining, and tracking changes in employment, prices, and other national economic measurements. In carrying out this mission, the DOL administers a variety of federal labor laws including those that guarantee workers' rights to safe and healthful working conditions; a minimum hourly wage and overtime pay; freedom from employment discrimination; unemployment insurance; and other income support. For more information, visit www.dol.gov on the Internet, and for poster information, see www.dol.gov/elaws/posters.hth.

Equal Employment Opportunity Commission (EEOC)

The Equal Employment Opportunity Commission (EEOC) protects the civil rights of those in the workforce through enforcement of various employment laws. Employers may not discriminate against employees based on race, sex, religion, national origin, physical disability, and age. For more information on the EEOC's application to small businesses such as medical practices, go to http://www.eeoc.gov/small/overview.html. The EEOC and employment laws are addressed in *Personnel Management of the Medical Practice,* Second Edition, ©2002 AMA Press.

CONCLUSION

Medical practice requires a lot of red tape to get started and has many rules and regulations to follow during the course of your professional life. This chapter will help you stay abreast of the requirements and assist you in staying on track. You are responsible for keeping informed of the issues and noting changes as they occur through announcements and bulletins as they are released by regulatory agencies.

chapter 5

Society Memberships/Practice Affiliations

INTRODUCTION

A medical practice is an enterprise that requires collaboration and coordination with other people and entities. Physicians need to be involved with other members of their profession and health care entities in daily scenarios, such as call coverage, medical staff privileges, sharing of services, referral patterns, as tenants in professional office buildings, and more. Managed care initiatives compel physicians to enter affiliations with other providers in organizations and relationships, such as independent practice associations (IPAs), individual practice organizations (IPOs), management services organizations (MSOs), and more. Further, most physicians desire to be involved in their communities in civic organizations as a way to contribute to their communities, to have a voice in local affairs, and to meet people. This chapter examines the benefits of memberships and affiliations for your practice.

MEDICAL SOCIETY MEMBERSHIP

Memberships in professional associations can benefit physicians throughout their careers, both individually and corporately, in the potential for exchange of information and in networking. Because of the multiple choices available and the considerable expense of dues, however, you should carefully consider what each organization has to offer and what its function will be for your practice. Not only will you have your own preference for what organizations to join, your practice will benefit from your staff members' attendance and participation in key professional affiliations and memberships. Membership in various medical societies, although not required for the practice of medicine, may be of benefit to the physician for the purpose of attaining information and networking. Moreover, associating your practice through these memberships will enable the practice to thrive by leveraging the resources often attained through these affiliations. Annual membership fees, in general, range from $100 to $1,000, or more. In the practice start-up phase, cash will need to be conserved; therefore, you will want to choose the affiliations that will be most beneficial for you and the practice. Payment of the dues is often a benefit of group practice or employment.

The following associations are worth consideration.

American Medical Association (AMA)

The *American Medical Association (AMA)* provides the physician a source of help and information about every aspect of the practice of medicine no matter where your practice is located. The AMA speaks out on issues that are important to patients and the nation's health. AMA policy on national health issues is decided through its democratic policy-making process—the AMA House of Delegates that meets twice a year. The House is comprised of physician delegates that represent every state; nearly 100 national medical specialty societies; federal service agencies, including the Surgeon General of the United States; and six sections that represent hospital and clinic staffs, resident physicians, medical students, young physicians, medical schools, and international medical graduates.

You do not have to be a member of the AMA to receive information or attend AMA-sponsored seminars. However, you will receive a discount on seminars, publications, and other services offered through the AMA if you are a member. The AMA is also an excellent source for continuing medical education (CME) and educational material.

National Specialty Societies

National and/or state specialty associations provide educational opportunities and information about particular specialties and allow you to interact with physicians who share the same specialty-specific concerns. Listed below are the organizations within the American Medical Association House of Delegates. To obtain a link on the Internet to *The Federation of Medicine,* go to the AMA website and click on:
http://www.ama.assn.org/ama/pub/printcat/1677.html.

To learn more about membership benefits, contact one of the specialty organizations listed in Table 5-1.

A list of names and addresses of professional associations can be found at the end of this book in Appendix A, Professional Associations.

State and Regional Medical Organizations

Table 5-2 is a list of state and regional medical organizations that are in the House of Delegates of the AMA. Because of state and regional issues, membership in these associations can be beneficial to the practice. For an Internet link to these websites, go to
http://www.ama-assn.org/ama/pub/printcat/7630.html.

Local Medical Societies

Local medical societies (ie, city and/or county) provide insight into the local concerns and politics of medicine and allow the physician

TABLE 5-1

The Federation of Medicine

Aerospace Medical Association
American Academy of Allergy Asthma & Immunology
American Academy of Child & Adolescent Psychiatry
American Academy of Cosmetic Surgery
American Academy of Dermatology
American Academy of Facial Plastic and Reconstructive Surgery
American Academy of Family Physicians
American Academy of Insurance Medicine
American Academy of Neurology
American Academy of Opthalmology
American Academy of Orthopaedic Surgeons
American Academy of Otolaryngology-Head and Neck Surgery
American Academy of Otolaryngic Allergy
American Academy of Pain Medicine
American Academy of Pediatrics
American Academy of Physical Medicine & Rehabilitation
American Academy of Sleep Medicine
American Association for Thoracic Surgery
American Association for Vascular Surgery
American Association of Clinical Endocrinologists
American Association of Electrodiagnostic Medicine
American Association of Gynecological Laparoscopists
American Association of Hip & Knee Surgeons
American Association of Public Health Physicians
American Clinical Neurophysiology Society
American College of Allergy, Asthma, & Immunology
American College of Cardiology
American College of Chest Physicians
American College of Emergency Physicians
American College of Gastroenterology
American College of Medical Genetics
American College of Medical Quality
American College of Nuclear Medicine
American College of Nuclear Physicians
American College of Obstetricians and Gynecologists
American College of Occupational and Environmental Medicine
American College of Physician Executives
American College of Physicians–American Society of Internal Medicine
American College of Preventive Medicine
American College of Radiation Oncology
American College of Radiology
American College of Rheumatology
American College of Surgeons
American Gastroenterological Association
American Geriatrics Society
American Medical Group Association
American Orthopaedic Foot and Ankle Society
American Psychiatric Association
American Roentgen Ray Society
American Society for Clinical Pathology
American Society for Dermatologic Surgery

TABLE 5-1 *Continued*

American Society for Gastrointestinal Endoscopy
American Society for Reproductive Medicine
American Society for Surgery of the Hand
American Society for Therapeutic Radiology and Oncology
American Society of Abdominal Surgeons
American Society of Addiction Medicine
American Society of Bariatric Physicians
American Society of Cataract and Refractive Surgery
American Society of Clinical Oncology
American Society of Colon and Rectal Surgeons
American Society of Hematology
American Society of Plastic Surgeons
American Thoracic Society
College of American Pathologists
The Endocrine Society
National Medical Association
North American Spine Society
Radiological Society of North America
Society of American Gastrointestinal Endoscopic Surgeons
Society of Cardiovascular & Interventional Radiology
Society of Critical Care Medicine
Society of Nuclear Medicine
Society of Thoracic Surgeons

to share ideas and information with other physicians who are practicing in the area.

Civic Groups

Becoming involved in local civic groups, schools, and other worthwhile organizations can benefit your practice indirectly and you personally, providing an opportunity to contribute to the community. Physicians often grow their practices by being known in the community in addition to establishing themselves based on their professional accomplishments. The more positive name recognition you can achieve, the more likely patients will be comfortable in seeking provision of health care from you.

OTHER PRACTICE AFFILIATIONS

Managed Care Organizations (MCOs)

In today's market, whether you are a participating or a non-participating provider in managed care often determines whether you are seeing patients. Therefore, considering affiliations with Managed Care Organizations (MCOs) is essential.

Once the address for the practice has been chosen, begin completing applications for participation in various managed care plans. The credentialing process is often lengthy and can take up to 60-90 days to process, so start early. It will be beneficial if you can begin to see managed care patients as soon as you open your office.

TABLE 5-2

House of Delegates of the AMA

Alabama
Medical Association of the State of Alabama

Arizona
Arizona Medical Association

California
California Medical Association

Colorado
Colorado Medical Society

Connecticut
Connecticut State Medical Society

District of Columbia
Medical Society of the District of Columbia

Delaware
Medical Society of Delaware

Florida
Florida Medical Association

Georgia
Medical Association of Georgia

Hawaii
Hawaii Medical Association

Illinois
Illinois State Medical Society
Chicago Medical Society

Indiana
Indiana State Medical Association

Iowa
Iowa Medical Society

Kansas
Kansas Medical Society

Kentucky
Kentucky Medical Association

Louisiana
Louisiana State Medical Society

Maine
Maine Medical Association

Maryland
Med Chi: Maryland State Medical Society

Massachusetts
Massachusetts Medical Society

Michigan
Michigan State Medical Society

Minnesota
Minnesota Medical Association

Mississippi
Mississippi State Medical Association

Missouri
Missouri State Medical Association

Montana
Montana Medical Association

Nebraska
Nebraska Medical Association

New Hampshire
New Hampshire Medical Society

New Jersey
Medical Society of New Jersey

New Mexico
New Mexico Medical Society

New York
Medical Society of the State of New York

North Carolina
North Carolina Medical Society

North Dakota
North Dakota Medical Association

Ohio
Ohio State Medical Association

Oklahoma
Oklahoma State Medical Association

Oregon
Oregon Medical Association

Pennsylvania
Pennsylvania Medical Society

Rhode Island
Medicine & Health Rhode Island

South Dakota
South Dakota State Medical Association

Tennessee
Tennessee Medical Association

Texas
Texas Medical Association

Utah
Utah Medical Association

Virginia
Medical Society of Virginia

Washington
Washington State Medical Association

West Virginia
West Virginia State Medical Association

Wisconsin
Wisconsin Medical Society

Regional Medical Organizations
Southern
Southern Medical Association

National
American Medical Association

Before attempting to participate in every plan available, do some investigative work. For example, specialists should ask the primary care physicians in the area what plans they belong to and which ones have the best reputation and the most patients. To receive referrals, participation in the same plans as the primary care providers is necessary.

If you are joining a group practice, discuss managed care participation with the medical director or office manager. The applications will most likely be completed for you. However, all necessary information to complete the forms must be provided. This information includes, but is not limited to, medical license, Board Certification, Drug Enforcement Agency (DEA) number, hospital participation, and malpractice insurance.

Be sure to read the section on managed care in Chapter 13, *Billing and Reimbursement Protocols,* before entering the managed care arena. You will also want to include your managed care affiliations in your marketing efforts so that patients and referring providers will know in which plans you participate.

Call Group Affiliation

A major hurdle in solo practice is finding other physicians in your specialty with whom to share call. Check with other physicians to see if there is an opportunity to join an existing call group. It may be necessary to take the initiative and start a new group. As a solo physician, look for every opportunity to share call with other physicians. Otherwise, there will be little opportunity for leisure or family time.

Physician Referral Service

Many hospitals have a physician referral service. Contact the local hospital(s) to see if such a service exists. Request to be added to the referral list for your specialty. These referral services often limit the number of physicians in each specialty. For this reason, it is best to start right away to sign up, or be put on a waiting list, if necessary. Ask whether they handle the referrals on a rotating bases or whether they give each patient a list of available physicians.

Emergency Room Coverage

Although the local hospital may have full-time emergency room coverage, opportunities may be available for you to work extra hours. If you are interested in *moonlighting,* contact the emergency room director at each hospital to see if such opportunities exist. If you are joining a group practice, check your contract to be sure there are no restrictions concerning employment outside the group.

CONCLUSION

Belonging to organizations that help you professionally is a wise move. Such organizations provide valuable resources and associations you will make. From interpretation of rules and regulations, to continuing education opportunities, to meeting local colleagues, you will most likely benefit from joining—and participating in—professional organizations at the local, state, and national levels.

Instituting Operational Procedures and Processes

INTRODUCTION

Medical practices today are facing an environment of ever-increasing complexity in patient management and third-party payment administration. To offset those complexities and reduce overhead costs, more practices are choosing to automate their processes through integrated billing, accounting, medical record keeping, and appointment scheduling. Computerized practices are generally more efficient and have better internal controls.

The arrival of managed care and increased overhead has made using computers in the medical practice not only helpful, but essential. The volume of reports and other statistical data requested by managed care organizations can only be handled aptly by a computerized practice management system. Developing a technology infrastructure and selecting systems will be discussed in more detail in Chapter 7, *Equipping Your Practice with Information Technology*. The purpose of this chapter is to discuss the operational procedures and processes to be instituted in your new practice, particularly establishing a fee schedule, purchasing supplies, and management of accounts payable.

ESTABLISHING A FEE SCHEDULE

There are various methods for establishing and reviewing fees in a medical office. The following are a few of those methods:

- Obtain fee information from other local practices in your specialty. It is important that your fees be comparable.
- Refer to publications such as *The Physician's Fee Guide* or *Annual Physician's Fee Reference Book* available in most medical bookstores.
- Use the Resource-Based Relative Value Scale (RBRVS) compiled by the Centers for Medicare and Medicaid Services (CMS).

The Medicare fee schedule has been based on the RBRVS system since 1992. Most indemnity insurers and managed care organizations are beginning to base their reimbursement on this system as well.

RBRVS in a Nutshell

The Resource-Based Relative Value system (RBRVS) is used to determine allowable reimbursement amounts and global days for surgery for Medicare Part B physician services. In the development of the RBRVS system, CMS (then HCFA) assigned a Relative Value Unit (RVU) to more than 7,000 Current Procedural Terminology (CPT) codes. For the complete and comprehensive history of RBRVS, visit http://www.RBRVS.com on the Internet. The site provides free downloads, such as RBRVS spreadsheets, formulas, and published Medicare data.

Each RVU has three components:

■ Work RVU
■ Overhead RVU
■ Malpractice RVU

When added together, these equal the total RVU.

Recognizing that the cost of practicing medicine varies in different parts of the country, CMS, then HCFA, assigned a Geographic Practice Cost Index (GPCI) to each component of the RVU for each CPT code.

Prior to 1997, the total RVUs were multiplied by a standard conversion factor to arrive at the allowable payment amount. Prior to 1997, Medicare has established a conversion factor for surgery, another for primary care services, and a third for nonsurgical services. Now there is one conversion factor, which is set at the following rate: The 2002 National Conversion Factors is 33.61992. See Figure 6-1 for the complete RBRVS formula.

With one standard conversion factor, this means all physicians in a given geographical area are reimbursed the same amount for a CPT code regardless of specialty.

NOTE: The Relative Value Units are reviewed annually.

FIGURE 6-1

The Complete RBRVS Formula

(Work RVU × Work GPCI) + (Overhead RVU × Overhead GPCI) +
(Malpractice RVU × Malpractice GPCI) × the conversion factor = Total Allowable

Example: CPT code 39502, Repair of a Hiatal Hernia, in Brownsville, Texas

Code 39502, Repair of Hiatal Hernia   Locality: Brownsville, TX

| $\dfrac{13.80}{\text{Overhead Work}}$ | $\dfrac{1.008}{}$ | = 13.841 |

| $\dfrac{12.57}{\text{Overhead RVU}}$ | $\dfrac{1.094}{\text{Overhead GPCI}}$ | = 13.751 |

| $\dfrac{2.58}{\text{Malpractice RVU}}$ | $\dfrac{1.025}{\text{Malpractice GPCI}}$ | = 2.644 |

Total RVUs for CPT 39502 in Brownsville, Texas = 30.236.

30.236 × 2002 conversion factor 33.61992 = $1,016.5319 (allowed).

Establishing your fees on the RBRVS system is the method of choice. Because CMS has already established the RVUs for each CPT code, using the Medicare fee schedule to establish your fees is very simple. However, you will want to increase the conversion factor or simply increase the Medicare fee schedule by 25 percent to 30 percent, depending on what other physicians in your area are charging for the same services and what other payers, such as Blue Cross, are paying.

For example, if a competitor charges $1,400 for CPT code 39502 (Repair of a Hiatal Hernia) and the 2002 Medicare Allowable for Code 39502 in your area is $1,016.53, the Medicare fee can be increased by 30 percent (approximately $300), and setting the standard fee at $1,325, while still be competitive in the area.

Cost of Providing a Service versus Practice Fees

However the fees are set, the practice cannot afford to deliver a service for a fee that is less than the cost of providing the service.

It is a fact that CMS took the cost of providing a service into account when it established the overhead RVU for each service. However, the CMS perspective of a reasonable profit margin may differ from a physician's, and it may not consider all the expenses in managing a medical practice. To maintain a practice that affords a reasonable profit/salary margin after the bills are paid, keep in mind the cost of supplies and other operating expenses. In time, expenses—with the exception of some variables—should be somewhat predictable. These predictable expenses are referred to as fixed costs. Figure 6-2 is an example of a breakeven chart that can be used to determine exactly what needs to be produced to exceed the breakeven point.

FIGURE 6-2

An Example of a Breakeven Chart

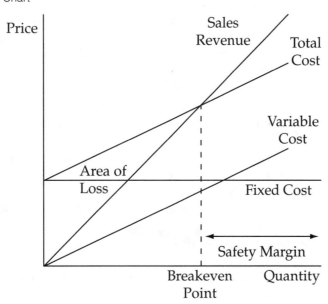

The secret to making a profit in business is knowing the fixed cost and variable cost. The fixed cost will not vary by adding additional output, but the variable cost may go up slightly.

For example, rent will stay the same whether the practice sees 10 patients a month or 100 patients per month, but supply cost will go up some with patient volume. With that said, profits will start the moment cost is exceeded, which is why it's important to know how much output (ie, productivity) must be achieved each day to exceed operating cost.

Case Study

A physician opens her office at 8:00 am. The daily fixed cost (eg, rent, staff, utilities) is $500 per day. The variable cost (eg, supply, repairs, overtime) is $150 per day. Her total daily cost is $650 per day. Her average reimbursement per patient (ie, output/productivity) is $62 per patient. Based on the above information, she needs to see 10.48 patients during the day to cover her operating cost before she can start paying herself. Depending on how many additional patients seen above the breakeven point will determine her compensation. Based on this study, if the provider wants to pay herself $150,000 per year, she will need to see an average of 20.48 patients per day and contain her cost to its current levels.

PURCHASING SUPPLIES

One of the routines that must be put into place in a medical practice startup to ensure that the practice is profitable is purchasing supplies. The first step in developing an organized purchasing system is to centralize the ordering process. Assign **one** person to be responsible for ordering supplies. In a new office, the Office Manager/Office Assistant should order supplies. Having one person in charge eliminates duplicate orders, adds objectivity, and prevents having sales representatives talk to more than one person. The employee in charge of purchasing becomes familiar with supplies and prices and thus can shop around for the best prices.

Centralized ordering will also allow the purchaser to establish the quantity of each supply used over a given time (eg, monthly). These usage guidelines allow development of an inventory process that will reduce unnecessary inventory and minimize the tendency to place panic orders that increase expenses.

Use a simple stenographer's pad as an order book or develop a form with the most common orders listed. Each employee who needs supplies or uses the last of the current inventory will list the item in the order book. The Office Manager will order supplies based on what is written in the book. Use of an order log or order sheets may also be established.

The following tips in Table 6-1 will help minimize the cost of supplies.

TABLE 6-1

Tips for Purchasing Supplies

1.	Create vendor files by company name and file all invoices and statements in chronological order. File the folders in alphabetical order.
2.	Be familiar with price breaks for regularly used items so that they can be ordered in quantities that provide the best price.
3.	Purchase office supplies at local office supply discount stores instead of ordering by telephone from an office supply business. This can save the practice up to 50% on some items.
4.	Every six months, check the prices on standard items and compare vendor prices. Ask for competitive bids from three different vendors.
5.	Ask for a 45-day payment window.
6.	Be aware of items being put on backorder. Never accept payment responsibility unless the order is received.
7.	Log all chemical orders on the Material Safety Data Sheet (MSDS) log.
8.	Negotiate for better prices!

ACCOUNTS PAYABLE

Practice operations include the accounts payable function, which encompasses writing checks, paying bills, and accounting for money spent. To set up a system for accounts payable, you may choose to purchase an off-the-shelf accounting package. Such packages are generally reasonably priced, will produce a general ledger, keep track of income, provide expense statements, and write checks. This is a viable option, particularly if the Office Manager already has experience with accounting software.

Practice management systems may also offer modules to handle the accounts payable function—usually at a higher price than off-the-shelf software. With the availability of reasonably priced software in the marketplace, however, it is unnecessary to forfeit any vital features of an accounts receivable package merely because it is offered. For example, you may see that it costs $2,000 to get an AP package with your practice management system, and you may think these need to be interconnected. If spending this extra money would cause you to forfeit a more important feature, such as on-line insurance verification, it is wiser to invest in the off-the-shelf software.

Most practices engage outside accounting firms to generate financial statements using output from the accounts payable and the accounts receivable information.

Chart of Accounts

The chart of accounts is simply a list of numbers that identify each category of expense in your practice by department. Your accountant will help establish a chart of accounts. Make sure the list is not too cumbersome. This information is necessary for the accountant to properly allocate expenses for tax purposes and cost accounting.

As an example, assume that the account number established for medical supplies is 105. A check is written to XYZ Supply Company for hypodermic needles. The check should be made out to XYZ Company in the proper amount, and the account number 105 should be noted on the check stub. This number tells the accountant that the check to XYZ was for medical supplies. For internal use, the invoice numbers that are paid should also be listed on the stub.

Correctly allocating expenses is essential to efficient practice operations. For accuracy, the person writing the checks—not the accountant—should be responsible for determining the account number to put on the check stub. The accountant may not know what supplies XYZ Company sells. Keep a copy of the chart of accounts available for ready reference.

Paying Bills

The accounts payment process works best if bills are paid only once each month. Unless a substantial discount is offered for early payment, never pay bills in less than 30 days from the date of purchase. Keep the money in the bank working for you as long as possible, not in the vendor's bank earning interest.

Pay bills from invoices, not from vendor statements. Vendors seldom have the same billing cycle you have. If payments are made from a statement, an invoice may mistakenly be paid twice. Most vendors will allow you to determine your invoice date.

At the same time each month, follow this routine outlined in Table 6-2 for paying bills.

Establishing a workable accounts payable system at the start of your practice is critical. Accurate tracking of supply costs reduces overspending and panic buying, provides information needed for budgeting and forecasting, and gives the accountant the information necessary to prepare financial statements and tax returns.

TABLE 6-2

The Payment Process

1.	Collect all the invoices that have been received from a vendor in the previous 30 days. Make sure that the person receiving the goods has initialed the invoice to show that all goods ordered were received and in the proper quantities. Total the invoices and write a check for this amount.
2.	Write every invoice number that is being paid and the amount on the check stub. Do not forget to put the chart of accounts number on the check and the check stub.
3.	Staple the invoices together, mark them *paid*, and write the date and check number on them. Buy a rubber stamp for this purpose.
4.	File the paid invoices in the vendor folder for that company. Keep only the invoices for the current year in the folder. At the end of each year, the invoices should be filed with other accounting papers for that year.

CONCLUSION

Medical practice is a business operation that requires the institution of certain policies and procedures to account for receivables and payables. Starting up a practice means that a fee schedule for services must first be established. Once that is in place, an accounting program and purchasing protocols can be set up. Consult with your accountant and health care consultant to ensure that you get off to a good start.

chapter 7

Equipping Your Practice with Information Technology

INTRODUCTION

With all the options available today, few can avoid being confused about what choices to make in equipping a medical practice with information technology. The purpose of this chapter is to present the fundamental options so that good decisions can be made about what is available and what will meet the needs of your practice.

USING TECHNOLOGY IN YOUR PRACTICE

The health care industry is often considered burdened with inefficiency and laced with labor-intensive processes to accomplish even a simple function. As practices continue to face these challenges, and with added pressure to their bottom lines, processes will need to improve for a practice to survive. Technology has revolutionized the world, yet most physicians still work in environments that rely on labor-intensive processes to perform their job. Even practices that have instituted technology improvements never realize the benefits because they fail to reengineer the processes around the technology.

As it has been stated so well:

"Automating a bad process not only ensures that we can do a bad job every time, but that we can do it faster and with less effort than before."

H. James Harrington, Business Process Improvement

To illustrate, Figure 7-1 looks at the typical workflow processes for pulling a single chart in comparison to working with electronic medical records. It shows that having data readily accessible without the hassles of manually searching for it has its benefits.

Case Study

It is 2:00 AM and the emergency room calls because a patient had an adverse reaction to the medication prescribed, and the patient does not recall the name of the drug. Will you remember? This is when a central database that stores all of your patient's medical records, accessible from home, would really come in handy. From the database you could e-fax or e-mail the entire chart to the emergency room if necessary.

FIGURE 7-1

Workflow Comparison for Paper Chart versus Electronic Medical Record

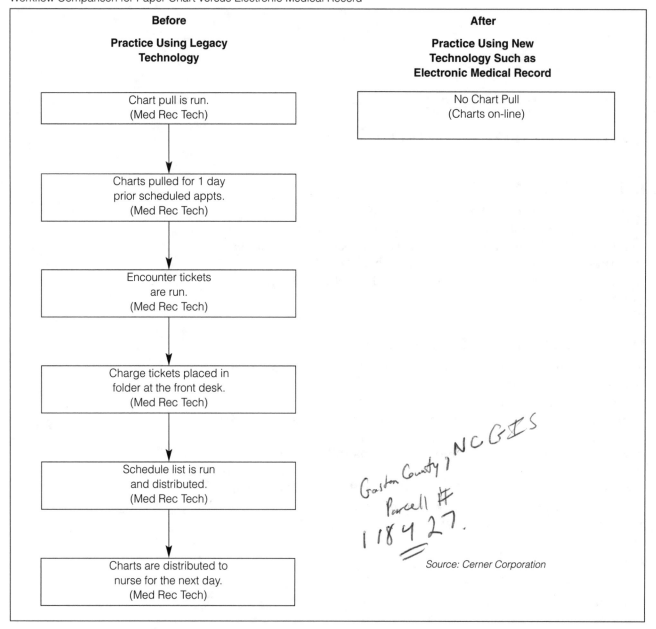

Source: Cerner Corporation

The Paperless Office

The previous case study may sound like *Star Wars* for the medical practice, but it is not. Many practices are achieving automated benefits through technology, including a totally paperless office and offices with fully integrated data repositories.

Although the benefits and possibilities are endless, costs are a consideration for any practice—especially at start-up when investment precedes revenue. For this reason building the technology infrastructure should be well-planned when you are starting a practice. The objective is to avoid cul-de-sac decisions that result in forced turnarounds, requiring the practice to rebuild at a later date to meet its needs and objectives.

In the beginning you will need to decide how you want to use technology in your practice. In today's market, it is easy to get distracted by the endless number of gadgets and vendors promoting their latest offerings. Moreover, some vendors will attempt to distract you with bells and whistles through dynamic power-point presentations without revealing the true functionality of the application. (Never take a vendor's word about how the application will work. Require them to show you a practice that is using their technology and that is accomplishing what you desire. Also, be sure to avoid the showroom sites.)

The goal of this chapter is to keep you from making the single most common mistake that many physicians make when purchasing technology—making a decision in a vacuum! This results in buying the wrong technology or over buying technology because "it would benefit the practice."

Just because you read an article or see a flashy demonstration of a vendor's product, or hear about a colleague's system, do not be quick to commit. Remember, the practice will be around for a long time. Be mindful of your investment and bear in mind all long-term goals and the economic ramifications of these decisions. Many of the solutions provided in today's market include hidden fees and reoccurring expenses that are often overlooked at the time of purchase. Consequently, you must do your research, and "let the buyer beware."

When building the technology infrastructure, consider the following factors:

1. **Cost.** While money drives many decisions, higher costs must be weighed against increased revenue and benefits. Select technology based on its ability to save you money and time. For example, should the practice spend thousands of dollars every year ordering encounter forms or superbills, or purchase a practice management system that will allow the practice to design and print its own forms at no cost. Or can the process be taken a step further and all charges captured electronically on a Personal Digital Assistant (PDA) [1] or Windows CE® device [2], and synchronizing it back into the billing module.[3] By taking this extra step or investing in a tool to eliminate the paper superbill and the charge entry process, operating cost is reduced.

---

[1] Personal Digital Assistant (PDA) is a handheld computer that serves as an organizer for personal information. It generally includes at least a name and address database, to-do list, and note taker. PDAs are pen-based and use a stylus to tap selections on menus and to enter printed characters. The unit may also include a small on-screen keyboard that is tapped with the pen. http://www.commweb.com/encyclopedia/search?term=PDA, 8/29/02.

[2] Microsoft CE® is Microsoft's personal assistant product.

[3] Data is synchronized between the PDA and desktop computer via cable or wireless transmission. http://www.commweb.com/encyclopedia/search?term=PDA, 8/29/02.

As a result, this approach would eliminate the encounter form altogether and the labor cost to key the charges. Moreover, the system would likely scrub the claim (ie, remove any errors or mistakes before it is sent to the insurance company to prevent costly denials) against your documentation to ensure that you remain in compliance, which is an immeasurable benefit, plus you will likely realize a higher level of reimbursement.

As noted, be mindful of hidden and/or reoccurring expenses, such as transaction fees, support fees, or future upgrades that can elevate the cost of the solution.

Following are hidden expenses that are often overlooked:

- Ongoing maintenance and support for hardware and software.
- Electronic transactions, such as electronic claims, insurance eligibility, remittance, and statements. Avoid arrangements that require a per-transaction fee unless the cost is justifiable.
- Future upgrades and new releases. Be advised that most medical software vendors will develop a new version every 12 to 18 months, necessitating continuous upgrades. Some vendors require their clients to pay for each new release. Other vendors include all continuous upgrades at no additional cost.
- Customization is almost always charged at an hourly rate of $100 to $200 per hour, depending on the requirements.
- Data conversions. Most vendors will charge from $2,000 to $5,000 to convert data from another system. (Vendors will almost always agree to negotiate on this fee to get the new business.)

Be aware of all reoccurring expenses—not just the initial sales price of the technology solution.

2. **Functionality.** While most functions are possible, in theory, one must be realistic. For example, some practice management systems incorporate rules into their processes, which are known as *rules-based systems*. A great tool, the rules alert the end-user before a mistake can be made. However, the rules must first be put into place and kept up-to-date before the benefits can be realized. Some systems allow the practice to link directly with the payers for obtaining eligibility and payer-specific rules. Do not just assume the rules come with the system.

Another functionality that can often be misleading is voice recognition. While this technology continues to improve, it generally requires months to train the application to become familiar with the user's voice. Even then, achieving 100 percent accuracy with this system is unlikely. When involved in a demonstration of voice recognition software, be mindful that presenters spend considerable time training their systems. Ask for permission to speak into the system yourself and you will instantly see a difference.

3. **Integrated versus Interface.** Integrated systems generally run on a single database with all of the functionality and workflow

converging through a single application. Integrated systems, which usually have lower licensing costs and do not require costly interfaces, are usually less expensive. However, if the integrated system cannot perform all the desired functions, it will require an interface to another application that would provide those functions.

Interfacing or combining applications (ie, known as the best-of-breed approach will allow buyers to build their perfect system. This approach is often used when specialized features are required or in the case of enhancing a legacy system, instead of replacing it altogether. The disadvantage of interfacing is having to deal with multiple vendors. This requires them to communicate with one another and, at times, share their technical expertise.

Methods for purchasing technology. Generally, there are three primary ways to acquire and maintain a technology infrastructure: (1) Standalone Systems, (2) Application Service Providers (ASPs), and (3) Web-based Systems.

Standalone Systems

Standalone systems, also known as the Client Server Approach, call for installing a central processing unit (CPU), or server, that will run the software application. Servers, which can be both local and remote, are connected to the other computers in the office by networking the workstations together

As an overview, the term *standalone system* simply implies that the application will reside on a dedicated server installed onsite at the practice. This approach will require the purchase of a software license and the necessary hardware to run the application.

The standalone approach is the most traditional and widely used. However, through the innovation of the Internet and virtual private networks (VPN), companies around the world are now offering alternative methods for delivering their information system (IS) solutions (discussed later in this chapter). The standalone approach is still a viable option, nonetheless, with its own advantages. Standalone systems are recommended to many practices, even after evaluating the alternatives, including ASPs. (See Figure 7-2, Client/Server Model, for a technical illustration of the standalone approach.)

The standalone system approach encompasses the following:
1. Select the vendors that will be needed to achieve the desired results. For example, the team of vendors compiled will consist of one with a practice management (PM) system, one with an electronic medical records (EMR) application, one with an appointment reminder application, and one for claims scrubbing. (Choosing a vendor for each application is called *best-of-breed selection*, which allows the building of the perfect

FIGURE 7-2

Client/Server Model

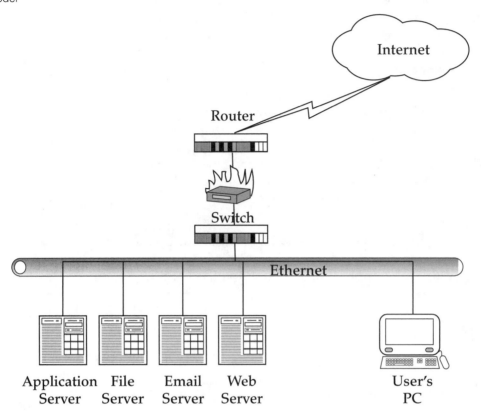

Source: The iLIANT Corporation

system. The total number of applications running together is optional.)

2. Agree on terms, maintenance cost, customization and consulting fees, support fees, future upgrade charges, and new software release expenses. In addition, consider recurring fees that include, but are not limited to, electronic data exchange (EDI) fees, electronic eligibility fees, statement fees, electronic payment posting, and supply costs.

3. Purchase the hardware that is needed to run the applications. If the PM, EMR, and e-mail are applied, likely there will need to be three servers plus an interface server to tie all the applications together. (Smaller practices generally require 1-2 servers.) The vendor should assist with this. Also, consider contacting an IS consultant for an explicit explanation of hardware requirements.

4. After installing the hardware, the applications will be ready for installation.

5. Once the applications are installed, the *databases and file queries* need to be built. This allows the system to be defined with resources and information specific to payers, referring providers, and charges. It will also be necessary to build payer profiles (formats) and to configure the EDI for electronic claims submission. (The vendor should assist.)

6. With a new system, allow for some testing and time to work out the bugs. Almost always, a new system will have some initial problems. (CAUTION: If applications combine by taking the best-of-breed approach, all the vendors will need to collaborate to resolve issues. This is often problematic with the installation of standalone systems that integrate to multiple applications.)

7. After inspection and testing, begin the training time, which will require 2 to 5 days.

8. Go live. (Begin using the system applications.) The average implementation time for a standalone system is 60 to 120 days from start to go-live, with the majority of the installations being completed within 90 days. For a comparison, this is an average of about 30 to 60 days longer than implementing an ASP. Therefore, if rapid deployment is necessary, the ASP approach would be more accommodating (see *The Application Service Provider (ASP) Approach,* discussed below.)

The advantages of the client/server approach are:

1. Practice owns the system
2. More control over functionality and interfaces
3. Ability to customize as needed (Most vendors charge $130 to $200 per hour for customization.)

The disadvantages of this approach include:

1. Ongoing maintenance
2. Bugs and glitches
3. Performance updates required
4. Hardware upgrades
5. Software upgrades
6. Recurring fees
7. Support fees
8. System administrative responsibilities
9. HIPAA responsibilities
10. Disaster protection and recovery responsibilities
11. Detecting and preventing intrusions

The Application Service Provider (ASP) Approach

Using an ASP is a lot like outsourcing transcription. Instead of hiring a full-time employee with benefits to transcribe dictation, the service is outsourced and the practice pays for the service by the line or word. With an ASP, you generally pay a fixed monthly hosting fee, and you outsource the system and all the maintenance and upkeep to the ASP. Below are the benefits of an ASP.

As an overview of the ASP Approach, an ASP is a company that will allow the use of its software applications on a subscription-based payment arrangement and deliver it in real time over an Internet connection or through a dedicated data communications line. Also known as *application hosting,* this approach allows practices to take advantage of powerful applications without having to purchase, install, and maintain them. Moreover, no substantial cash outlay is required and deployment can be rapid because the system is already developed and running.

The ASP approach includes the following:

1. Select an ASP that offers the software applications and services that are desired.
2. Agree on terms. (The fee is fixed and there is nothing to buy; thus, the process is straightforward.)
3. Establish connectivity. (This can take 30 days or more and varies by location.)
4. Determine the number of workstations and users needing to access the system.
5. Determine if any data conversion or migration is required.
6. Connect a dedicated data communications line or virtual private network (VPN) to the ASP's data center. (The ASP will handle this for you.)
7. Application is turned on and training started one to five days after connectivity.
8. Two to five days of training.
9. Go live with new ASP.

The average implementation time for an ASP, from start to go-live, will average from 30 to 60 days, with the majority of the installations being completed within 40 days after the line is installed. If necessary, the system could go live within one day of installing the line, but users will need training and the database will require some customization.

Because the telephone service provider is responsible for installing the line, installations that are delayed generally result from scheduling issues.

Advantages of the ASP approach can be summarized as follows:

1. Software is never outdated (always on the most current version).
2. All upgrades and new releases included.
3. All support included.
4. System maintenance and upkeep provided.
5. Interfacing provided and supported.
6. Access to industry experts (IT experts).
7. No major hardware required (low capital investment).
8. Subscription base pricing (pay as you go).
9. No unexpected fees (monthly fixed amount).
10. Minimum cash outlay.
11. Less out-of-pocket expenses.
12. Disaster protection.
13. Data redundancy and data mirrors.

14. HIPAA compliant.
15. Future IS compliance standards handled by the ASP.
16. Eliminates the challenge of procuring and implementing complex systems.
17. Access to information anywhere in the world.
18. Eradicate capital expenses, maintenance fees, supporting, and upgrading fees.
19. Transferring the responsibilities of managing the application, thus enabling practices to focus on patients.
20. System is already developed and ready for rapid deployment.
21. Assures customer an ongoing return on investment. Because the system is *rented*, the customer can cancel the subscription when it is deemed no longer a benefit to the practice (subject to contractual terms and conditions).
22. An array of applications from which to choose.

Some examples of the disadvantages to the ASP approach are as follows:

1. Connectivity required (additional expense)
2. Optimal performance contingent on bandwidth speeds
3. Customization and interfacing subject to the ASP's approval
4. Control imposed by the ASP and may limit some functionality
5. Data stored off site
6. Loss of control
7. The stability (ie, instability) of the ASP

The cost for a single provider can range from $1,500 for basic billing application with limited functionality to $100,000 for a fully integrated EMR system on a wireless network with interfaces to outside entities, such as the hospital, lab, and radiology. However, the average price for a good practice management system for a single provider with four users will range from $25,000 to $60,000 (hardware included).

Application service providers are usually less expensive when analyzed over a five-year period. For example, an ASP will charge a monthly hosting fee that generally ranges from $200 to $800 per month per provider and includes the following services:

- Complete practice management system
- Continuous upgrades at no additional cost
- Internet access
- Routine system backups
- Disaster recovery
- 24-hour security protection
- 24-hour data protection
- Technical and user support
- Training
- Ongoing system maintenance

FIGURE 7-3

ASP Client Model

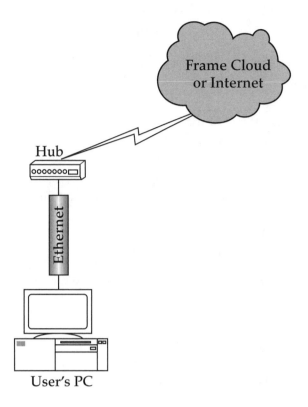

Source: The iLIANT Corporation

Figure 7-3 is an illustration of the ASP Client Model.

Internet/Web-based Application

Practice management applications delivered over the Internet are similar to the ASP approach, except they are considered by some experts to be less secure and connectivity can be less reliable. Applications delivered over the Internet offer providers an economical opportunity to get started without a major investment.

Other considerations before investing are the history of the application and the vendor's stability. Products and vendors are in and out of the marketplace without regard to their customers who sometimes are left without solutions and recourse. In current-day vernacular, if a vendor *sunsets* (ie, discontinues) an application or goes out of business, you will have what is referred to as an *orphan* application. Over time the application will become outdated and the resources to support it will be unavailable. Spend time researching each vendor and their references. Request a site inspection, but be cautious to avoid the vendor's showroom sites. Vendors will often offer inducements to their showroom sites that refer them business.

If you are considering EMR, it is recommended that you shadow a physician in a live clinical setting to experience the tool first hand while it is in use.

SELECTING THE RIGHT KIND OF TECHNOLOGY

Follow the guidelines below for selecting the information technology that is right for your practice:

1 Start with a plan. (ie, How will the technology be deployed?)
   a. Standalone server
   b. Application service providers
   c. Web-based applications
2. Set objectives and criteria. (If with a group, develop a committee.)
   a. Know your deal breakers
   b. Understand the economic ramifications
   c. Know the return on investments
   d. Understand the reoccurring fees
3. Follow a disciplined evaluation process for each vendor.
   a. Request for Information (RFI)
   b. Request for Proposal (RFP)
   c. Controlled Demonstrations
   d. Pre-selected criteria for qualifying and disqualifying the vendors
4. Develop a long-term technology plan
5. Develop a partnership understanding with the vendor
6. Insist on superb support and service
7. Understand the agreement and contract
8. Insist on a walk-away clause or an amenable dispute resolution clause

PURCHASING YOUR SOLUTION

Buying technology is a lot like playing with building blocks. To begin, a few basic components are needed. As the infrastructure is built, each component must continue to work with the original components. Also be mindful that technology is a fluid process that continues to evolve and advance, which calls for carefully considering the purchasing options. Following are some options for purchasing technology.

- Buy a turnkey system. Thousands of vendors sell turnkey systems that have everything needed for a technology infrastructure packaged together (ie, hardware, software, installation, training, and ongoing support). Turnkey systems generally use off-the-shelf software that is widely used by other medical practices. Turnkey systems are the most common method employed for buying technology for a medical practice; however, over time it can be expensive to maintain and support. Turnkey systems are also known for having recurring costs and hidden fees.

- Build your own system. Some vendors will sell their application out of the box and allow you to install the system yourself. These systems are often less expensive because the vendor has less responsibility and less availability. Computer savvy physicians who are experienced in IS should only consider this option. The cost advantage can be considerable; however, the commitment is extensive. Moreover, you will need to be knowledgeable in IS with the ability to troubleshoot your own problems.

■   Outsourcing through an ASP/BSP. As noted earlier in this chapter, the process of securing your technology objectives through an ASP is straightforward. The ASP will require a contract of 3 to 5 years, with agreed terms lasting the life of the contract. Typically, an ASP will offer two levels (or tiers) of contracting. With one company, for example, the first level will include application hosting as well as other services, with a general cost of $400 to $600 per provider per month depending on the number of providers. There is also one initial implementation fee of $2,500 to $7,500 or more for large health systems (depending on the number of providers). The second level includes the first tier of services plus the ASP's professional services (ie, billing and collections, payment posting, accounts receivable management, insurance filing and follow-up). Reporting can also be obtained for a percentage of net collections. The percentage can vary depending on specialty and volume.[4]

CONCLUSION

Become an informed purchaser from the start-up of the practice. Resist the temptation to buy too much, too soon, before knowing the practice's objectives. Consider various options, research vendors thoroughly, and tap into the resources of trustworthy consultants before you over—or under—invest in technology solutions. Let the buyer beware!

---

[4] For more information, contact the iLIANT Corporation at www.iliant.com or (813) 855-6880.

chapter 8

Identifying Insurance Requirements

INTRODUCTION

Among the most crucial decisions to make for the practice includes the purchase of various types of insurance coverage. Due to the many liabilities inherent with the practice of medicine, protecting yourself through insurance will be a vital reality of running your practice. State law requires every physician to carry some types of insurance; other types of insurance are required by your hospital or managed care plans; and still others are a result of financing your office or equipment leases. Additionally, you will need to decide what level of risk you are willing to take and what protections are financially feasible. For example, will you insure small losses that you might incur, or do you accept the risk and absorb replacement cost—and at what level.

Knowing what to protect is another concern. For example, a patient who trips on loose carpet and falls at your office door may sue you, even if you lease office space in a medical building. (See Chapter 14, *Loss Prevention and Risk Management*, for more information of developing a risk management plan.) If the fall occurs within your suite, you, not the landlord, may be at fault.

Every medical employer carries some form of insurance in addition to professional liability coverage (ie, malpractice). This might include property insurance, commercial general liability insurance (CGL), life insurance, overhead disability insurance, Workers' Compensation insurance, group health insurance, and fidelity bond insurance that protects the practice if there is embezzlement. The purpose of this chapter is to address the many questions about insurance that arise in a practice start-up and direct you to the appropriate resources to answer your needs.

PROFESSIONAL LIABILITY INSURANCE

Professional Liability Insurance, or medical malpractice insurance, is available through various sources, including traditional insurance companies, physician-owned companies, self-insured companies, group purchasing programs, and risk retention groups. What is available to you depends largely upon how much coverage you plan to purchase and the vendors who are in your area. Not all carriers operate in every state.

Depending upon your specialty, professional liability insurance may be the single highest expense, but it will be the most important insurance you can buy. According to The Doctor's Company, a national malpractice carrier owned and operated by physicians, there are 17 claims filed each year for every 100 full-time practicing physicians. For high-risk specialties, the number of claims is higher. As a result, according to Richard E. Anderson, MD, Chairman for the Doctor's Company, some physicians are practicing defensive medicine to avoid liabilities, which is a violation of the Hippocratic Oath.

Choosing a Professional Liability Carrier

Aspects to consider when choosing a carrier for medical malpractice insurance include the following:

- Company's financial condition. Because litigation takes 3 to 5 years, seek coverage from a company with financial stability that is apt to be around to defend you.
- Risk management/loss prevention assistance and advice. Concurrent with conducting risk assessments of your practice, your liability carrier should be a resource for training, education, and guidance for your staff in implementing loss prevention measures that strengthen the practice.
- A comprehensive policy. Make sure you know what your policy covers and does not cover. Review a copy of the policy, paying particular attention to the exclusions.
- Experienced claim professionals and a strong legal network. Just as you would research any professional you hired, research and scrutinize prospective malpractice carriers by checking references and evaluating credentials.

Purchasing Coverage for Malpractice Claims

Consider the following points when purchasing medical malpractice coverage:

- Purchase adequate limits. Many physicians purchase coverage based on the minimum requirements of the hospital(s) in which they practice, usually $1,000,000 per occurrence and $3,000,000 aggregate. However, a single occurrence can exhaust the coverage under an existing policy. The aggregate should be two to three times the occurrence limit.
- Understand the claims-made coverage and the importance of continuous coverage. A distinction exists between claims-made coverage and occurrence policies from continuous coverage. Some insurers deny the renewal of existing policies or refuse to set the cost of tail coverage for future claims based on incidents that have occurred during the policy period. If the policy term is one year, then the insurer is free to modify the policy at the end of that term. If the policy is continuous in nature, the insurer cannot unilaterally modify its terms. The policy period is shown on the declarations page of the policy.

- The added expense of higher limits of liability. Consider whether they may be cost effective for you or not.

- Name your professional corporation on your policy. Because most legal actions will name both you and your corporation, be sure to name a professional corporation on the policy.

- Consider insuring the corporation separately. By considering insuring the corporation separately, available coverage can be increased for a fraction of the cost of increasing your individual limits.

- Make sure that professionals are properly covered. Office professionals, such as nurses, professional assistants, nurse practitioners, or midwives, in your employ should be properly covered through their own coverage.

- Check with provider about discounts. Ask if they give a discount for using an electronic medical records system.

NOTE: If you are joining a medical group, most likely the group's policy will cover you. The premiums may be a part of your compensation package. If you already have malpractice coverage that you will cancel when you join the group, you will need to purchase tail coverage (malpractice insurance that covers you in the event of future claims on past acts) to cover any potential litigation stemming from actions prior to the new group coverage taking effect. [1] Be sure you check with the new group/employer to find out who is responsible for payment of premiums for tail coverage. Leave nothing to chance!

BUSINESS INSURANCE

Certain aspects of office management and equipment must be covered by insurance to provide financial protection. One way to purchase the protection that is needed for your practice is to buy a professional office package (POP). Insurance for a medical practice should include general liability, business contents, property (if you own your building), umbrella liability, business auto, computer, employee dishonesty, business interruption insurance, and equipment breakdown coverage.

Commercial General Liability Coverage (CGL)

The CGL policy is a comprehensive form of coverage that provides protection from lawsuits brought against you by third parties. A third-party person is any individual other than the policyholder, the insurance company, or persons specifically exempted from coverage under the policy. The policy typically includes personal injury, product liability, advertising liability, and contractual liability. Look for policy limits of $1,000,000 to $5,000,000. The cost for the higher limits is often minimal.

---

[1] Anderson RE. The billions for defense: The pervasive nature of defensive medicine. The Doctor's Company Website. http://www.thedoctors.com/Resources/Articles/defensivemed.htm. 03/10/02.

You will also want to consider non-owned and hired automobile liability coverage for damages to a third party by an employee's vehicle used for the business of the practice, such as going to the bank or post office. This coverage would include damages to a third party incurred by an employee using rented automobiles while working on behalf of the practice.

Property Insurance

A considerable amount of money has been spent to purchase the furniture and equipment necessary to start your practice. Evaluate the cost to replace the tangible assets owned by the practice to determine the proper amount of insurance to purchase. Purchase an adequate amount of property insurance to replace fixed assets in the event they are destroyed by fire or another disaster. In addition, include office supplies, medical supplies, medical books and journals, artwork, files, and file contents.

You may purchase many options through your property insurance. Depending on locale, you may want to consider earthquake or flood coverage, which are usually excluded from property policies. Always request *special* or *all risk* coverage. Consider higher deductibles to reduce costs. For reliability, try to use companies rated "A" or better by A.M. Best.

Computer Coverage

Your property insurance will likely cover the computer hardware; however, you may wish to purchase additional coverage that includes loss due to power surges or loss of data. Consult a software vendor to see how much software insurance is needed for the practice's licensed software.

Business Interruption Insurance

Business interruption coverage, which is important and inexpensive, is somewhat like disability insurance for your office. If your office becomes inaccessible due to a covered property loss (eg, fire, hurricane, etc), this coverage will reimburse you for lost revenue, continuous expenses, and lost profit. Be sure that the coverage includes funds for a temporary office, expediting expenses, advertising the new location to your patients, and the expenditures to move back into your office once the damages are repaired.

Employee Dishonesty Insurance

This coverage protects your practice from losses due to employee theft or embezzlement of funds.

Equipment Breakdown Coverage

This insurance covers the cost to repair or replace equipment that may be a means of generating significant revenue to your practice. Coverage also includes lost revenue for the period that the equipment is unusable.

Umbrella Policy

In addition to the standard office package, you may want to consider an umbrella policy, which provides comprehensive catastrophic coverage for claims beyond the normal limits of the regular policies. These policies generally start at a million dollars coverage and go up from there.

WORKERS' COMPENSATION INSURANCE

Workers' compensation insurance is mandatory in most states if you have three or more employees. Each state regulates benefits and costs so most policies have identical coverage. Make sure the policy you purchase is covered by your state's insurance insolvency fund.

Premiums are based on payroll estimates for a 12-month policy term, subject to a final audit to adjust for changes. All wages should be included in the payroll estimates, including bonuses. Overtime, however, may be adjusted to its regular time equivalent, rather than the time-and-a-half wage rate.

Inquire about the following when purchasing workers' compensation insurance:

- Insurer's provider network.
- Safety program discounts.
- Caps for offers (which can offer big savings). Some states do not require owners or principles of a business to cover themselves under workers' compensation plans. Because premiums are based on wages paid by the practice, a substantial sum can usually be saved by not covering yourself. This is only advisable, however, if you already have a good disability policy and health insurance plan in place.

PURCHASING INSURANCE POLICIES

Following are other guidelines for purchasing insurance products:

- Higher deductibles usually mean lower premiums.
- Avoid over buying. Expensive *add-ons* are unnecessary if you have good coverage on your basic policy.
- Select appropriate policy limits and buy larger amounts of protection when it is economical. Increasing your limits under a liability policy is usually cheaper than adding coverage under a second policy.
- Self-pay smaller claims, adhering to legal parameters. Consult with your insurance advisor or plan on this option.
- Give prompt attention to any third-party claim.
- Pay premiums annually instead of monthly. Typically, an annual payment is less expensive than monthly installments.

Whatever the type of insurance coverage you purchase is no substitute for risk management. Work with your insurance agent to help you develop a sound loss prevention program for all forms of practice liability. Conducting a regular loss prevention in-service education program will keep your employees aware of the importance of loss prevention and on-the-job safety.

Review your insurance program regularly. Read your policies and confer with your insurance agent or consultant (and with legal counsel, as appropriate) regarding your insurance program. Policies differ, needs differ, costs vary—a sound insurance program to achieve adequate protection of corporate and personal assets requires careful and continuous review.

The checklist in Figure 8-1 is an Insurance Plan Assessment that will help assess your insurance plan and protection.

FIGURE 8-1

Insurance Plan Assessment

A. Property—Building—Consensus

1. What perils are you insured against?
   - ■ Fire, extended coverage, and vandalism.
   - ■ Sprinkler leakage, if needed.
   - ■ All risk, including burglary and theft.

   Is coverage on a:
   - ■ Replacement cost basis—no deduction for depreciation?
   - ■ Actual cash value, subject to depreciation?

   What is:
   - ■ Deductible?

		Yes	No
2.	Is coverage limit adequate to comply with coinsurance clause?	Yes	No
	Does coverage for contents include coverage for building items installed at your expense and in which you have an insurable interest until lease expires?	Yes	No
	If building coverage is provided, is there any exposure to loss due to condemnation after a fire loss due to nonconforming construction? If so, is policy properly endorsed?	Yes	No
3.	Review exposure and policy coverage for outdoor signs and awnings.	Yes	No
4.	Are the named insured and lien holders properly designated on the policy?	Yes	No

B. Time Element

1. Is business interruption or loss of earnings covered?   Yes   No

2. What perils are you insured against?
   - ■ Fire, extended coverage, and vandalism.
   - ■ Sprinkler leakage, if needed.
   - ■ All risk, including burglary and theft

   Is coverage on a:
   - ■ Replacement cost basis, no deduction for depreciation?
   - ■ Actual cash value, subject to depreciation?

   What is:
   - ■ Deductible?

		Yes	No
3.	Is coverage limit adequate to comply with coinsurance clause?	Yes	No
	Does contents coverage include coverage for building items installed at your expense and in which you have an insurable interest until lease expires?	Yes	No
	If building coverage is provided, is there any exposure to loss due to condemnation after a fire loss due to nonconforming construction? If so, is policy properly endorsed?	Yes	No
4.	If building is owned, is rental income coverage carried?	Yes	No
5.	Is extra expense insurance carried?	Yes	No

Insurance Plan Assessment

C. Separate Floaters			
1.	Is glass coverage required and carried?	Yes	No
2.	Is accounts receivable records coverage carried?	Yes	No
	In absence of coverage are records properly protected in a fire-resistant safe or cabinet and/or are records duplicated and kept off premises?	Yes	No
3.	Is there any fine arts coverage?	Yes	No
4.	Is there any valuable papers and records coverage to cover cost or research and development necessary to reproduce records destroyed?	Yes	No
5.	Is data processing coverage needed?	Yes	No
6.	Do lease requirements of leased personal property require "all risk" floater insurance?	Yes	No
7.	Are instruments, cameras, or other equipment scheduled for specific off-premises coverage?	Yes	No
D. General Liability (Excluding Professional)			
1.	Is coverage on a comprehensive form?	Yes	No
2.	Is coverage included for personal injury, including suits involving employment?	Yes	No
	Is coverage provided without participating in loss?	Yes	No
3.	Is coverage provided for liability assumed under contract?	Yes	No
4.	Is coverage provided for fire, legal liability for leased premises?	Yes	No
5.	Are special extensions or coverages required for owned or non-owned watercraft or aircraft?	Yes	No
6.	Host liquor (not sale) liability coverage?	Yes	No
7.	Additional insured employees?	Yes	No
8.	Products?	Yes	No
9.	Independent contractors?	Yes	No
E. Auto Liability and Physical Damage			
1.	Are all owned autos insured for:		
	■ Liability—bodily injury and property damage?	Yes	No
	■ Medical payments?	Yes	No
	■ Uninsured motorists?	Yes	No
	■ Collision?	Yes	No
	■ Comprehensive?	Yes	No
	■ Towing and replacement auto?	Yes	No
	■ Is special coverage required for installed radio receiving/transmitting equipment?	Yes	No
2.	Is coverage provided for the liability of employee vehicles used on your behalf or hired vehicles through a non-owned and hired auto endorsement?	Yes	No
3.	What are deductibles for comprehensive and collision coverage?	Yes	No
4.	Is an endorsement necessary to make corporate-owned vehicle coverage as broad as a personal policy?	Yes	No
F. Excess Umbrella Liability (Excluding Professional)			
1.	Is coverage carried?	Yes	No
2.	Is limit adequate?	Yes	No
3.	Do underlying policy (Items D and E) limits meet umbrella requirements?	Yes	No
4.	Is coverage provided on a first dollar defense basis for those suits not covered by underlying policy?	Yes	No
5.	Any special exclusions that require further explanation?	Yes	No
G. Crime			
1.	Is employee dishonesty coverage carried with adequate limit?	Yes	No
2.	Is employee dishonesty coverage carried or required by ERISA-1974?	Yes	No
3.	Is coverage required for other crime areas?	Yes	No
	■ Money and securities on and off premises?	Yes	No

FIGURE 8-1 *Continued*

Insurance Plan Assessment

■ Depositor's forgery?	Yes	No
■ Credit card forgery?	Yes	No
■ Contents burglary and theft if not provided under Item A?	Yes	No

H. Workers' Compensation

1. Is coverage required and carried?	Yes	No
2. Are certificates of insurance requested for all independent contractors performing work in your behalf to prevent additional premium charges?	Yes	No
3. Any loss frequency or severity that indicates problems, and are you receiving company engineering assistance?	Yes	No
4. Does policy cover employee injury in other states?	Yes	No
5. Voluntary compensation exposure?	Yes	No
■ Sponsored athletic groups exposure?	Yes	No

I. Boiler Coverage

1. Is coverage required for explosion of steam or hot water boiler?	Yes	No
2. Is coverage on a replacement cost basis—no deduction for depreciation?	Yes	No
3. Is limit adequate?	Yes	No
4. Is coverage provided for other boiler exposure areas such as:		
■ Business interruption or loss of earnings?	Yes	No
■ Rental value?	Yes	No
■ Extra expense?	Yes	No
5. Is coverage required for other machinery exposures, particularly if you are the owner of a building, such as but not limited to:	Yes	No
■ Air conditioning equipment?	Yes	No
■ Electrical switchboards?	Yes	No
■ Transformers?	Yes	No
■ Unfired pressure vessels?	Yes	No
■ Electric motors?	Yes	No
■ Compressors?	Yes	No

J. Miscellaneous: Have exposures been examined for the following areas of coverage?

1. Fiduciary responsibility insurance?	Yes	No
2. Directors and officers liability—for own corporations and boards on which you may serve?	Yes	No

K. Make sure the agent reviews ISO (Fire Rating Bureau) inspection reports for rate surcharges due to correctable property conditions.

Source: *The Business Side of Medical Practice*, pps. 53-57, American Medical Association, 1989, Chicago, Illinois.

CONCLUSION

Buy the insurance that is needed—whatever the practice scenario—to protect both the practice and yourself from exposure to liabilities and to meet legal requirements. Get help from a trustworthy advisor and work closely with a reputable insurance agent or broker to make good decisions to limit your exposure to loss.

Financing the Medical Practice

INTRODUCTION

The average physician completes residency with an accrued debt in excess of $100,000. Now consider that most new start-up practices can operate for as long as 3 to 4 months and without any substantial cash flow to support operations. Even practices once owned by hospital networks or physician practice management companies (PPMCs)—with a track record of profitability—that are considering venturing into private practice are apt to experience lag time in terms of cash flow.

Situations like these call for some kind of financing or infusion of start-up capital. This is nothing out of the ordinary; all sizes of entities borrow cash every day for new ventures that cannot be sustained without some kind of outside help. Not only will cash be needed until the practice can support itself, but some kind of initial investment will be necessary to purchase tangible items and equipment required.

Without personal wealth or other sources of funding, the capital (ie, money) needed to start and sustain a medical practice will have to be obtained from an outside source. At some point in the start-up stage, financing or a line of credit will have to be established.

The purpose of this chapter is to discuss the process of obtaining adequate financing for starting a medical practice.

FINANCING OPTIONS

Paradoxically, virtually anyone—with or without a decent credit history—can secure a reasonable amount of money to buy a car or a house, but the money to start a small business, especially a medical practice, can be a little more scarce.

First, when physicians try to procure capital to start a practice, they face two common problems: (1) usually, they are leveraged extensively and carrying a high debt load as result of 12 years of additional education; and (2) medical practices have very little tangible assets—or collateral—to back up this debt. The physician's greatest asset is knowledge, and as great as this may be, a bank cannot repossess *knowledge* in the event of default on a loan.

Not all banks are reluctant to lend money. Plenty of lenders are willing to loan money to physicians, although you may need to look a little harder to reach your dream of a successful, private medical practice. Often times—especially in smaller towns—lending money to a new physician is a great public relations tool. In other cities, banks have organized special small business loans, which again are great public relations tools for banks and something in which physicians should take advantage.

The Small Business Administration (SBA) is another source. This federally funded program does not actually lend money, but it does guarantee the lender that the loan will be repaid in full. However, you do have to work with an institution that belongs to the SBA (most larger banks do); and as a government program, the paperwork can be burdensome.

Lenders that specialize in one specific field, such as health care, are another option for financing a start-up. While these *boutique* lenders are viable options to traditional sources of capital, using them can be expensive. Finance charges and services received from boutique lenders are typically at a premium and thus should be resorted to only after all other options have been exhausted.

Conversely, specialized lenders in health care are likely to be more understanding of a physician's needs, and, thus should not be overlooked. Keep in mind that when a traditional institution, such as a bank, is reluctant to lend you money because you are asking for a large amount of unsecured credit, the boutique lender may be more willing to listen.

Most boutique lenders have more leeway to work with physicians with flawed credit. Further, a boutique lender may offer the perfect opportunity to a physician who is highly leveraged with their original lender, but needs a little additional cash flow to make ends meet.

It is good to know that there is someone out there who is willing to help a struggling physician. Bear in mind, though, while boutique lenders are ready and willing to work with a physician in a tough financial situation, they require a higher return on their investment for the additional risk involved. Even though it may cost a little more, it may certainly be worth it in the long run.

THE PRO FORMA

Before you can even think about walking into a bank or some other lender and asking for a line of credit, you must have some sort of financial projections. If professional help was attained to develop a business plan for the practice, the work will likely encompass pro forma financial projections. Though, in most cases a full business plan is unnecessary at this stage, and the pro forma alone will suffice.

A pro forma is a projection. It is a compilation of data based on reasonable assumptions as to the performance of an entity. A very useful tool, a pro forma is used to forecast the operating results of a practice (or any other entity).

Recently, pro formas have received somewhat of a bad name because of their misuse by public companies. Certainly misuse is a possibility, but when correctly used within their operating parameters, the pro forma can be an excellent planning and budgeting tool (though, it is technically not a budget by the strictest of terms).

Any lending institution that a physician approaches regarding starting a line of credit will require the physician to have some sort of projection of how the business will perform. In addition, the institution will almost always insist that an independent third party develop the financial projection (ie, someone with no interest in how the business performs).

A pro forma is no different from the financial statements of any other company. It usually contains a detailed profit and loss statement (ie, income statement) and a statement of cash flow. What makes this document unique, however, is the fact that all of the information contained in these statements has yet to occur. This is why, in addition to these statements, the pro forma must contain detailed information concerning the assumptions used to create the statements. Without this data, the profit and loss statement and statement of cash flow are meaningless.

This is why it is integral to this process to have someone knowledgeable in the operations of a medical practice help create such a document. Remember, these lenders are about to give you a sizeable amount of money—usually anywhere between $150,000 and $200,000 for a single provider—so they want to know all of the details. How and when you plan on making money, how and when you plan on spending the money, and, most importantly, how and when you plan on paying back their money.

The pro forma consists of two main categories: revenues and expenses. Certainly, anyone can write down a revenue number and an expense number, but the acid test is whether they are realistic figures, and is their sufficient documentation to support the conclusions. If not, the pro forma is worthless.

While the pro forma should be accurate and realistic, it is still a projection, and projections can—and will—vary from the actual results. The best tool in developing a pro forma is common sense. If it does not look right, then it probably is not.

As said before, a pro forma can be divided into two categories: expenses and revenues. With some detailed analysis as to the type of practice, the services that will be offered, and a myriad of other issues, these two can be accurately hypothesized.

For instance, the staff that will be needed is fairly predictable. Salary ranges for employees in the area are generally attainable. Add a percentage for benefits (ie, retirement plan contribution, health and dental insurance, etc) and get a pretty good idea of what the total employee salary expense will be. Now, do this for every other expense that is incurred in a medical practice and the job will be half done.

Next, consider revenues. Through extensive research, determine the average reimbursement per visit, or surgery, or whatever may apply for your specialty. Decide on the number of patients per day that you can see, remembering to be realistic. Multiply the two and you will know the average revenue per day.

If it were this easy, of course, anyone could build a pro forma, but unfortunately it is not and they cannot. In fact, a great deal more analysis is involved before even the first statement can be produced.

For instance, to be as accurate as possible, the physician(s) will want to know or at least have a good idea what equipment will be needed. For the most part—depending on the specialty—most of the tangible items will be similar from practice to practice. Every practice needs items such as exam tables and secretarial chairs and waiting room chairs, and knowing this is very important to the preparation of the pro forma. This equipment will likely be the biggest single cash outlay by the practice. This is why it is best to determine exactly what each physician wants and does not want before the pro forma is developed. A sample provided in most initial questionnaires is included as Figure 9-1. This encompasses a list of the most general medical and office equipment that a practice will need to operate.

FIGURE 9-1

Pro Forma Initial Questionnaire

Medical Equipment	
Quantity	Description
	Adult scale
	Anesthesia machine
	Aspirator
	Audiometer
	Autoclave
	Biohazard trash hamper
	Blanket warmer
	Bronchoscope
	Cautery unit
	Chlestech LDX Lipid Profile System
	Colposcope
	Defibrillator
	Digital thermometer
	Doppler
	Double-lock narcotics cabinet

FIGURE 9-1 *Continued*

Pro Forma Initial Questionnaire

	EKG machine
	EKG stand
	Electrosurgical generator
	Endoscopy
	ENT wall unit
	Exam stool X 4-6
	Exam table X 4-6
	Eye chart
	Handheld cobalt blue light
	Handheld pulse oximeter
	Hematology analyzer
	Infant scale
	IV poles
	Laparoscopic video system
	Liquid nitrogen tank w/ ladle
	Mayo stand
	Medical lighting
	Microdermabrasion system
	Microscope
	Midmark spin stool
	Ophthalmoscope
	Otoscope
	Outpatient exam light
	Pelvic light
	Procedure table X T
	Pulmonary function unit
	Pulse oximeter
	QuickVue influenza test
	Scale
	Sphygmomanometer X 2
	Spirometer
	Sterilizer
	Stethoscope X 2
	Thermometer X 2
	Two-section X-Ray viewbox X 2
	Tycos stethoscope
	Tympanometer
	Vision screener
	Vital signs monitor X
	Wall unit sphygmomanometer
	Wheelchair X 2
	X-Ray machine and processor X T

Office Furniture/Equipment	
Quantity	Description
	Bookcase
	Break room chair
	Break table
	Waiting room chair
	Coat rack
	Coffee table

F I G U R E 9-1 *Continued*

Pro Forma Initial Questionnaire

		Copy machine
		Couch
		Credenza
		Credit card machine
		End table
		Executive chair
		Executive desk
		Fax machine
		Filing cabinet
		Floor lamp
		Large refrigerator
		Manager's desk
		Medical record cabinet
		Parsons table
		Point side chairs w/o arms
		Printers
		Reception desk
		Safes
		Secretarial chair
		Step stool w/ handle
		Table lamp
Appliances/Equipment		
Quantity		Description
		Bottled water machine
		Coffee maker
		Extension cords/surge protectors
		Flashlight
		Mail meter
		Microwave
		Outdoor combo ashtray
		Refrigerator (large)
		Refrigerator (small)
		Soda machine
		Telephone system
		Toaster oven
		Tool box
		Trash cans
		Typewriter
		Video player and monitor

Once the foundation of expenses and revenues has been established, they can be used to construct the profit and loss (ie, income) statement and the statement of cash flows. If these statements are going to be used to procure financing or a line of credit, the committee that reviews this information will not only look at the basis from which it was formed—the assumptions—but it will also look at the manner in which it has been presented. This is why the profit and loss (ie, income) statement and statement of cash flows should be prepared in accordance with Generally Accepted Accounting Principles (GAAP). This will ensure that while the person reviewing the pro forma will have never seen it before, they will be familiar with the manner in which it has been created.

CONCLUSION

Procuring a line of working capital or financing for the start-up of your medical practice should not be harder than your board exams! This may not be quite as easy as it once was due to the lagging economy, but there will always be people out there who are willing to lend someone money for a reasonable business venture. Even if your credit is less than stellar, someone will be more than willing to provide you with the financing you need.

Remember to be prepared though. Most lenders are not going to lend someone $175,000 just on your good name. They are in their business to make money, and they need some proof that time and effort has been invested and the proper amount of research has been done to make this venture work. The pro forma is a must when applying for a line of credit.

The pro forma is an intricate document prepared by someone knowledgeable in both the health care field and in finance. The basis for the numbers used—their assumptions—are as important as the numbers themselves. And without proper documentation and supporting evidence, the pro forma can potentially do more harm than good.

Selecting and Leasing Space and Purchasing Equipment

INTRODUCTION

Among the many decisions involved in starting a medical practice is where to set up the office and how to furnish and equip it. Your specialty, practice style, and locale will have a lot to do with your choice of office space. Access to capital will be a major factor in the choice of furnishings and fixtures, as well as office equipment. The purpose of this chapter is to review the variables that need to be considered in order to make lasting decisions that are beneficial to the growth and function of your practice.

SELECTING AN OFFICE LOCATION

The type of practice you will be establishing is the progenitor of the office site you will select. Choosing a geographic area that is in line with your specialty is critical to the success of the practice. For example, an obstetrician will need to have easy access to a hospital in order to attend patients and deliver babies, while a pediatrician may need to locate in the suburbs where he or she is accessible to families with children.

In addition to geographic location, it is important to know exactly what you want or do not want in a lease before you start looking. For example, how much space will actually be needed and how much space will be needed to sustain the growth of the practice. Several Internet websites offer the ability to calculate square footage requirements for office space by inputting information about your business. One such site is www.officefinder.com. OfficeFinder, a national organization that provides assistance to tenants, recommends the considerations listed in Table 10-1 be reviewed prior to beginning the office location decision process.

Negotiating a Favorable Lease

Location, not cost, should be the determining factor in an office lease. Remember that a lease is a binding agreement; you may be locked in for several years. Also, leasehold improvements and other concessions can be negotiated up front.

TABLE 10-1

Office Space Planning Checklist
___

Features:
- Best three features of current space
- Worst three features of current space
- Most important features

Timing:
- Occupancy date
- Time line for process

Location:
- Geographic location
- Access

Budget/Cost:
- Budget and cost

Site Accessibility:
- Freeway access
- Public transportation

Layout Type:
- Offices versus open work areas

Employees:
- Number
- Sizes of offices and work areas
- Windows
- Special needs

Lease Options:
- Expansion
- Extension
- Termination
- Contraction
- First right of refusal on adjoining space

Reception Area:
- Seating
- Upgrades

Work Areas:
- Types
- Sizes
- Equipment
- Special electrical needs

Lease Length:
- Lease length
- Extension options

Growth Projections:
- 3 year
- 5 year
- 10 year

General Feel:
- Spacious or efficient
- Lighting quality

Conference Rooms:
- Seating capacity
- Number
- Image
- Public/private

TABLE 10-1 *Continued*

Security:

- Building
- Neighborhood

Amenities:

- Lunch rooms
- Coffee bars
- Lounge
- Rest rooms

Parking:

- Number on site
- Total required
- Cost

Mechanical Systems:

- Elevators
- HVAC
- Off-hours operation

Identity:

- Signage
- Visibility

Image:

- Type of building
- Location in building
- Location on floor
- View
- Building and floor size
- Quality of improvements

Source: *Office Space Planning Checklist.* http://www.officefinder.com/checklist.html. 08/29/02.

How much you are able to negotiate on the lease rate varies with supply and demand. For example, if ample office space is available, negotiating an excellent deal is highly possible. Conversely, if only limited office space is available, the landlord will be much less willing to negotiate.

Set priorities for the items that are important to you in the contract and seek advice from an attorney before you sign. Obtain everything about the leasing arrangements in writing. Make no agreements based simply on a verbal assent, regardless of who the landlord will be. A well-written lease protects both the lessor and the lessee.

What to Look for in an Office Lease

Below is a list of some considerations in office leasing that are most important to physicians:

- **Know Your Timeline.** Making a decision on the right space and location can take weeks or even months.
- **Know the Description of Your Space.** Be sure to understand how the space is being measured; then personally measure it. Hallway space is sometimes included in the square footage. Do not pay for space that cannot be used, especially common areas such as a lobby or foyer that is shared with other tenants.

Check to see if the rental agreement includes parking spaces. Find out how many and where they are located. If patients have no place to park, the office space is useless. A good rule-of-thumb measure is one parking space for every chair in the reception area.

- **Know Your Terms.** We recommend that you sign a first lease for no more than three years. This will allow enough time to give the locale a fair chance. A viable practice should begin to show strong profits by the third year. While a 10-year lease may feature an attractively low rent, getting out of it may be hard if you decided to move to another location.

- **Know Your Renewal Options.** As an alternative to a long-term lease, consider signing a 3-year lease with two 3-year options to renew. These options should include any future rental increases in writing.

- **Know Your Rental Terms.** Know to whom the rent is payable. A landlord who lives halfway across the country is not likely to be as responsive to your requests for repairs and improvements as one who lives in the same town.

- **Know Your Escalation Clause.** Even a 3-year lease may have rental increases every year. These increases are usually based on the landlord's taxes and cost of operations, such as maintenance and utilities. Rent in commercial space is quoted as cost-per-square-foot annually.

- **Know Your Damage Deposit.** Find out how much damage deposit is required and if your deposit will earn interest. Be sure that all repairs are made before move in or that an appropriate clause noting the needed repairs is included in the lease. Most leases have some wording concerning the condition of the space after the lease has expired. Some will state that "all leasehold improvements become the property of the landlord," or "the premises must be returned to their original condition." In either case, the tenant loses. You will either give up items you have installed, such as sinks, cabinets, wallpaper, and even expensive draperies; if not, you will have to resurface and repaint the walls. This can be very expensive if you decide to move.

- **Know Your Escape Clause.** Be sure that the office lease contains an escape clause releasing you from your obligations should you lose your license, hospital privileges, or become disabled. An escape clause should also be included to protect your estate in the event of your death.

- **Know the Items and Services Furnished.** Maintenance, security, repairs, lawn mowing, and snow removal all fall into this category. Make no assumptions about anything. Any services furnished and costs covered must be itemized in the lease. Check out the credentials of the building maintenance service and be sure they are bonded. If you plan to see patients at nontraditional hours, be sure you know the hours of operation for the air conditioning, elevators, and security. Be clear about the kind of signage that is allowed or provided.

- **Know What Type of Insurance Is Provided by the Landlord.**
  Learn what kind of coverage the landlord has for accidents that
  may occur in the foyer, parking lot, and so forth. Check with an
  insurance agent to see if a supplemental policy is needed for any
  gaps that may exist.

- **Know the Terms for Remodeling and Redecorating.** Does the
  lease agreement state how often your office will be repainted or
  the carpet replaced? How often does the landlord repaint or
  redecorate the common areas? Who pays for these
  improvements?

- **Know the Terms for Subleasing.** If you choose to move before
  your lease expires, will you be allowed to sublet your space?
  Does the lease restrict the sublet clause to certain kinds of
  businesses? While you want the sublet clause to be reasonable,
  you also want to assure that another tenant does not sublease
  space to an undesirable tenant.

- **Know Your Unfit-for-Occupancy Clause.** This clause usually
  covers storm damage and other acts of nature. However, you
  will want to assure that the lease covers other disruptions such
  as loss of heat or air conditioning. You may not be able to see
  patients for several days, and you want to be sure you do not
  have to pay rent for those days the space is uninhabitable.

- **Know Your Rights of First Refusal.** This clause states, "You will
  be offered the first opportunity to lease any additional space that
  becomes available in your building." If your practice grows
  rapidly, you will want this option to expand rather than relocate.

Chapter 9, *Financing the Medical Practice*, lists the basic pieces of
furniture and equipment necessary to start up a medical practice. In
the following pages are discussions about leasing office equipment,
medical devices, and furniture.

ACQUIRING EQUIPMENT

Acquiring equipment calls for a knowledge base that many
physicians may not possess. However, the following information
may help with the decisions. Consider the advice of an accountant
and a trustworthy health care consultant to prevent overbuying or
overspending.

Leasing versus Purchasing

Before acquiring equipment items, discuss with your accountant the
advantages of leasing versus purchasing equipment. Leasing entails
higher interest rates, but requires lower down payments. Generally,
because of limited access to capital in a practice start-up, highly
technical equipment should be leased rather than purchased. Most
vendors will offer the option to lease equipment, and most leasing
companies will offer several leasing options. After the purchase
price is established, your accountant will calculate and advise you
on the best way to attain the item, based on the capital that is
available, current interest rates, the technology of the equipment,

and total cash investment requirements of the practice start-up. Leasing also allows you to diversify your debts and it does not tie up your working capital.

Another option for obtaining a lease is to utilize a leasing consultant/broker who will shop around for the best rate. Leasing consultants have helped many physicians acquire all of their purchases through a single lease, instead of obtaining a separate lease for each purchase. Along with the convenience of making one payment, consolidating financing arrangements into a single lease will likely achieve a lower overall finance rate.

For certain types of equipment, leasing may be a viable option when considering what the equipment will be worth in five years. For example, a computer selling for $2,000 today will be outdated in five years and worth $150. With a lease, you would just turn the equipment back to the leasing company at the end of the term and replace it with a new computer, and continue with the lease. Following are some examples of equipment that is often leased.

Telephone System

When it comes to buying equipment, vendors will often oversell on bells and whistles, when all that is really needed is functional equipment—often the case when it comes to telephone systems. For example, some vendors will attempt to sell you the top-of-the-line system, with features that will rarely be used. *Selling short* is another method vendors will use to take advantage of consumers. Vendors will sell you equipment without informing you that additional apparatuses may be required or that the system will be outgrown in a year, giving them assurance of having you as a repeat customer for upgrading equipment. For these reasons and because outgrowing equipment is quite common, especially for new businesses, leasing is often considered. Leasing offers the convenience of not having to own equipment that requires replacing every so many years.

Because the telephone system will be a vital link between you and your patients, knowing and buying the right system will be critical. *Key systems* are mostly common for small businesses because they do not need a lot of features. Key systems are also inexpensive— much less expensive than a Private Branch eXchange (PBX), an in-house telephone switching system that interconnects telephone extensions to each other as well as the outside telephone network. Another leading-edge consideration is PC-based telephones (telephone software that resides on the personal computer). These systems can offer all the features of the large systems at the price of a key system. A good resource for telecommunications and buying tips for telephone systems and PC-based systems can be found at www.commweb.com, which offers product reviews, buying guides, and case studies.

Medical Devices

You will likely be adding expensive medical devices that, like telephone systems, can become obsolete with the advances of newer more efficient technology and equipment. Various tools used in medical practice include electrocardiographs, laboratory and diagnostic equipment, laser devices, radiology equipment, etc. Some companies offer a full line of equipment for the convenience of not having to contact a separate vendor for each device. To enhance their attractiveness and convenience, these vendors may also offer financing or leasing arrangements. Be extremely cautious, however, before adding any medical devices to the practice before knowing if third-party payers will reimburse for services performed using these devices.

Another option for obtaining equipment is to consider purchasing or leasing pre-owned or refurbished devices that can still be under a manufacturer's warranty. Inquire about closeout or demonstration models, which are often sold at a discount. It is important to maintain a low overhead when starting out by not adding a lot of expensive equipment until you establish the patient volume to support the added expenses. Doing so will allow you to cost-justify the purchase before going into debt over a piece of equipment that will likely be outdated before its revenue-generating potential is optimized.

Copy Machines

Leasing a copy machine with a good service contract is a wise decision. Copiers are relied upon extensively. They are complex machines with hundreds of moving parts and require ongoing maintenance. Owning one can be expensive, especially when considering the cost of ownership over the life of the copier. Therefore, leasing a copy machine is a popular solution. There are many leasing programs to be considered, but be cautious of the commitments that are made. For example, some agreements may offer attractive terms, but the agreement may obligate the leasee to purchase copier supplies exclusively through one vendor. In many instances, supplies from such vendors are two and three times more expensive than prices offered at local office supply stores.

Also, know the performance level of the copier that is being considered. Copiers will almost always have a three- or four-digit model number. The last two digits indicate the number of copies per minute (CPM) that the machine will generate. While so many copies per minute may seem insignificant, consider the amount of nonproductive time the staff will spend standing at the copier. Also compare the warm-up speed, the reset speed, and the initial copy speed. Then compare performance to cost.

Fax Machines and Printers
Unless you are using high-end printers and fax machines, you may discover that purchasing is more economical than leasing this equipment since cost of ownership is somewhat less expensive and the equipment is low maintenance. For example, a business fax machine will retail for approximately $150 to $200. If it ever needs to be replaced, it is more economical to purchase outright rather then paying a monthly lease payment for several years.

Computers
In Chapter 7, *Equipping Your Practice with Information Technology*, the options are discussed for deploying and acquiring technology, which entails the purchase of computer hardware to run the system. Regardless of what deployment method is selected for delivering technology, you will need to purchase some type of computer hardware. The application service provider (ASP) approach will require the least amount of hardware to be purchased, but still some hardware will be required. Many physicians who are just starting out see the purchase of a computer as a key step in the right direction. However, it is recommended that, before rushing out to buy an expensive computer, you determine the overall hardware requirements within the practice's global information system strategies. Otherwise, a computer may be purchased that is not compatible with the long-range plan. When it comes to leasing computer hardware, we are finding that more physicians are opting to purchase their system because computers have become much more affordable, especially pre-owned units that are being sold for $100 to $300.

Be cautious of any software vendor that discourages you from buying your own hardware. In many cases the software vendor will go out and buy the equipment from the same places you could buy it, but mark it up 10 to 20 percent before reselling it to you. Some vendors will require you to use their preferred equipment because of their software and support requirements, but you should still be allowed the option of buying your own hardware.

Furniture
Leasing furniture is also an option, but for a practice starting out, buying used furniture may be a better choice. The market is flooded with used furniture and it is fairly common to find all matching pieces. Moreover, furniture in the waiting room will receive its share of abuse; therefore, new furniture will soon look old after a few months of heavy use. Artwork and other decorative items can also be added without excessive expense if you know where to look.

Another cost-saving option is to buy new furniture for the home and bring the old furniture to the office. For example, perhaps the kitchen table at home would make an excellent table for the breakroom at the office. If you are going to buy a new table anyway, why not buy one for your home and bring your old table to the office. To add some atmosphere to the office, you may want to consider setting up the waiting room like the living room of a home and adding home decorations throughout the office such as table lamps, coffee tables, bookshelves, and other comfortable and charming pieces that remind people of home. This will make the office more inviting and less intimidating.

When it comes to buying or leasing assets, there are plenty of options to consider. You may be able to buy everything at once if you find a fully furnished office or a practice that has recently closed. Regardless of the direction that is chosen, it is extremely important to stay within your budget, especially during the initial months of starting the business. Keep in mind that it can take up to 90 days before any revenue is generated and up to 1 to 2 years before the revenue stream is fully realized. For this reason, your overhead, including your personal draw (salary), must be considered before adding layers of expense.

CONCLUSION

Selecting an office space and engaging in a lease arrangement and negotiations are some of the most confusing aspects of a start-up. Purchasing equipment, furniture, and fixtures for your practice can be mind-boggling, as well. Most of these decisions are long-lived and expensive. Seek help from your attorney, accountant, and a health care consultant who has the practice's best interest in mind and experience in working with others in similar circumstances.

chapter 11

Managing Personnel

INTRODUCTION

An overview of the essentials of personnel management is presented in this chapter. As an employer, the physician starting in medical practice must know quite a bit about labor and employment laws that govern all businesses in addition to knowing about customary compensation and benefits. Further, employers have responsibilities and standards that are a part of management.

Even as an employee, a physician is viewed as an authority figure in a medical practice. The clinical assistants and administrative staff expect the physicians to understand and follow the rules. If you plan to become an employee of a group practice, hospital, or other entity, you should have a working knowledge of the laws and statutes regulating the medical practice, and a thorough understanding of the internal personnel guidelines that pertain to managing the employees.

EMPLOYMENT LAWS

Employment laws are the rules and regulations that form the basis for managing personnel. Written to protect the rights of the workforce, upon these principles rests the relationship between employer and employee.

Employment discrimination laws seek to prevent discrimination by employers based on race, sex, religion, national origin, physical disability, and age. Discriminatory practices include bias in hiring, promotion, job assignment, termination, compensation, and various types of harassment. Employment discrimination laws are embodied in federal and state statutes, both in the private and public sector.

Resources are furnished at the end of this chapter that will give extensive information concerning employment laws.

Title VII of the Civil Rights Act of 1964

Title VII, which applies to employers with more than 15 employees who work 20 or more hours per week, prohibits discrimination on the basis of a protected status such as race, color, religion, sex, national origin, or physical or mental disability in regard to hiring, termination, promotion, compensation, job training, or any other term, condition, or privilege of employment.

Sex includes childbirth or related medical conditions. The Pregnancy Discrimination Act forbids employers from discriminating against workers on the basis of pregnancy, childbirth, or related medical conditions. Women affected by pregnancy must be treated in the same manner as other applicants or workers with similar disabilities or limitations, such as temporary medical conditions. For additional information, refer to: http://www.aflcio.org/rightsatwork/disc_pregnancy.htm.

Sex discrimination is defined as unwelcome conduct, whether verbal, visual, or physical, that is based on an individual's protected status, and that results in a tangible employment action, or that is severe or pervasive enough that it unreasonably interferes with an individual's work performance, or creates an intimidating, coercive, hostile, or offensive environment. The most common form of harassment is sexual harassment.

The Nineteenth Century Civil Rights Act, amended in 1993, ensures all persons equal rights under the law and outlines the damages available to complainants in actions brought under the Civil Rights Act of 1964, Title VII, the Americans with Disabilities Act of 1990 (ADA), and the Rehabilitation Act of 1973.

Age Discrimination in Employment Act (ADEA)

Both Title VII and the federal Age Discrimination in Employment Act (ADEA) prohibit employers to discipline or discharge an employee who is more than 40 years of age because of age. The ADEA contains explicit guidelines for benefit, pension, and retirement plans. The ADEA does not regulate job-related discipline.

Americans with Disabilities Act of 1990 (ADA)

The ADA, which is broader than outlined by Title VII, protects persons with disabilities from discrimination in employment, public services, public accommodations, and telecommunications. The statute has two components that affect the medical practice. The first one pertains to discrimination in hiring or employment and requires an employer to make reasonable accommodations for an employee with a disability if he or she can perform the essential functions of the job. The second component pertains to accommodations that must be provided for persons with disabilities to access your facility or services. These accommodations, for example, would include having a wheelchair ramp or a restroom that is large enough to accommodate a wheelchair.

Fair Labor Standards Act of 1938 (FLSA)

Administered by the Department of Labor, the Fair Labor Standards Act (FLSA) regulates workers' time and money. This law defines the 40-hour workweek; sets minimum wage (eg, currently $5.15 per hour), restricts child labor, and sets requirements for overtime pay. The FLSA applies to all employers whose annual sales total $500,000 or more or who are engaged in interstate commerce—a legal requirement so broad that it includes those who make telephone calls and send mail from one state to another.

Most FLSA violations occur because employers misunderstand the rules controlling which workers are covered and must be paid minimum wages and overtime for any hours over 40 that they work each week.[1] (Employment classifications are defined later in this chapter.)

Equal Pay Act

The Equal Pay Act, which amended the Fair Labor Standards Act in 1963, prohibits paying wages based on sex. It provides that where workers perform equal work in jobs requiring "equal skill, effort, and responsibility and performed under similar working conditions," they should be provided equal pay.

Rights of Military Personnel

The Uniformed Services Employment and Reemployment Rights Act of 1994 (USERRA) prohibits employment discrimination on the basis of an individual's membership, applying for membership, or serving in the military. USERRA covers all employees who perform military service, either voluntarily or involuntarily, including active duty, training for active or inactive duty, and full-time National Guard duty. Employers may not take any of the following actions on the basis of military service or obligations:

- Deny initial employment
- Deny reemployment
- Terminate the employee
- Fail to promote the employee
- Fail to provide the employee any benefit of employment

If military service was a factor in the decision to take any of these actions, the employer must prove that the action would have occurred anyway to avoid charges of discrimination.

Discrimination for Sexual Orientation

Though not a part of federal law pertaining to civil rights, there is a growing body of law preventing or occasionally justifying employment discrimination based on sexual orientation. Employers should check with their state governments to see if there is legislation against discrimination for sexual orientation.

---

[1] Repa, BK, The FLSA: The Law of Time and Money @2000 HR One. Available at: http://library.lp.findlaw.com/scripts/getfile.pl?FILD-legpub/hr/hr000002&TITLE=Subject&T. 08/10/2001.

Workplace Privacy

Privacy is a person's right to keep personal information away from the world at large—the right to be left alone. However, an employee's desire for personal privacy may conflict with an organization's need to collect employment-related information and act upon it. Increasingly, employers are being held responsible for workers' conduct during the employment relationship and sometimes for prehire conduct an employer should have discovered. For protection, employers are searching workspaces and electronic documents, running credit checks on potential hires, and requesting detailed medical information. The law allows employers to use information obtained in a credit and background check for employment purposes, but requires employers to inform applicants, within three days of the request, that an investigation report has been requested.

The US Constitution does not grant a right to privacy on workers in private companies, but other provisions give some workers such rights. Basically, the ADA and the Family and Medical Leave Act (FMLA) protect a worker's health status (ie, employee medical records). That is, the worker's health records must remain confidential and separate from the employee's personnel file.

Other relevant legislation to protect the privacy of the applicant or employee are the Fair Credit Reporting Act (FCRA) and the Electronic Communications Privacy Act (ECPA).

Equal Employment Opportunity Commission (EEOC)

The Equal Employment Opportunity Commission (EEOC), established by Title VII of the Civil Rights Act of 1964, interprets and enforces the Equal Pay Act of 1963, Age Discrimination in Employment Act of 1967, Title VII, and Title I of the Americans with Disabilities Act.

EMPLOYMENT CLASSIFICATIONS

Part of the practice's responsibility when hiring the practice staff encompasses obtaining a working knowledge the Fair Labor Standards Act (FLSA). This complex law determines whether an employer is subject to federal minimum wage and overtime requirements. Most medical employees are covered. For compliance, first ascertain the status of your practice. Then, conclude the exempt or nonexempt status of each employee using the descriptions below.

Exempt Status

The following employment categories have been adapted for application to the medical practice for defining employees who are exempt from overtime pay requirements. These categories include:

- Executive Employee. Employees must meet all of the following definitions to be exempt (eg, practice administrators are typically considered exempt)
  - Minimum salary—$155 per week
  - Primary duty—manages enterprise, department, or department subdivision
  - Other job characteristics
    - Directs the work of two or more full-time employees
    - Exercises discretionary powers
    - Authorized to hire and fire or to recommend those actions
  - Must spend no more than 20 percent of working hours in nonexempt duties
- Administrative Employee. Employees must meet the following definitions to be exempt (eg, administrative assistants, personnel directors, office managers, and laboratory supervisors are typically considered exempt):
  - Minimum salary $155 per week
  - Primary duties:
    - Office or nonmanual work
    - Work relates directly to management policies or general business operations
    - Works directly in academic instruction or training
  - Other job characteristics:
    - Uses discretion and independent judgment regularly
    - Assists owner, executive, administrative employee
  - Must spend no more than 20 percent of time in nonexempt duties
- Professional Employee. Employees must meet all the following requirements to be exempt (eg, physicians, registered nurses, registered or certified technologists, physician assistants, speech pathologists, and physical therapists are typically considered exempt):
  - Minimum salary $170 per week
  - Primary duties—work requires advanced knowledge acquired through specialized study of an advanced type in a field of science
  - Other job characteristics
    - Must consistently exercise discretion and judgment
    - Intellectual in nature
  - Must spend no more than 20 percent of workweek on activities unrelated to professional duties

Nonexempt Status

Common medical practice positions that typically are considered *nonexempt* are:

- Licensed practical nurses

- Nurses' aides
- Laboratory technicians or assistants
- Clerical workers
- Orderlies
- Food service employees
- Janitorial employees

WAGE RECORDS REQUIREMENTS

The FLSA requires that employers keep records on wages and hours worked. Wage records should include the following for each employee:

- Full name as used in Social Security Administration records
- Social Security Number, employee number or symbol, as used in payroll records
- Home address, including ZIP code
- Date of birth, if the employee is under the age of 19
- Sex
- Position title
- Time of day and day of week employee's work begins
- Regular hourly rate of pay
- Amount and type of pay for any pay that is not included in regular rate
- Hours worked by employee on each work day and total hours worked for week
- Employee's total daily or weekly earnings (not including any premiums paid for overtime)
- Employee's total payment of overtime for the workweek
- Total wages for employee for each pay period
- Date of each payment made to the employee and pay period covered by the payment
- Total amount of additions to or deductions from wages for each pay period
- For each deduction, the employer must show the date, amount, and nature of the deduction

Unless the employee is exempt from overtime pay, the employer must pay one-and-one-half times the employee's regular rate of pay for all time worked over 40 hours in one workweek. Even if an employer pays every two weeks, there can be no *averaging* of hours in the pay period. For example, if the employee works 30 hours the first week of the pay period and 50 hours the next week, he or she is entitled to 10 hours of overtime pay for the second week. Overtime is based on hours *worked* over 40, not including vacation and sick leave taken during the same pay period.

AT-WILL CONTRACTS

The most common type of employment agreement in the health care industry is the oral, *at-will* agreement. The concept is that an employee can quit at any time, or the employer can terminate the employee at any time, with or without reason.

At-will does not apply to a job in which a contract is in effect stating a specific period of employment. The right of the employer to apply the at-will doctrine does not override the restrictions placed on the employer, such as the discriminations defined in Title VII of the Civil Rights Act of 1964.

By using the term *at-will* versus *just cause*, an employee serves at the discretion of the medical practice and therefore may be dismissed with or without cause. Using the term *just cause* sets a prerequisite that justifiable cause must be shown in order to discharge an employee. The practice's employee handbook (discussed later in this chapter) should use specific language indicating that employees of your practice are employees at-will.

POSTING REQUIREMENTS

Federal and state laws often require employers to post a notice about a particular law. Usually provided as posters or permits, these notices should be in a conspicuous place easily accessible to all employees (eg, typically, the breakroom). Listed below are the posters that employers are required to display under federal law.

Age Discrimination, Disability Discrimination, Equal Employment
- Poster titled *Equal Employment Opportunity is the Law*
- Available from national or regional EEOC offices or on the Internet at: www.dol.gov/esa/regs/compliance/posters/eeo.htm.

Child Labor, Minimum Wage, and Overtime
- Wage-hour poster 1088 (Federal Minimum Wage)
- Available from the US Department of Labor poster office and regional offices or on the Internet at: http://www.dol.gov/esa/regs/compliance/posters/pdf/minwagebw.pdf.

Family and Medical Leave
- Poster required by Family and Medical Leave Act of 1993
- Available from the US Department of Labor poster office and regional offices or on the Internet at: www.dol.gov/esa/regs/compliance/posters/fmla.htm.

Polygraph Testing
- Wage-hour poster 1462 (Employee Polygraph Protection Act)
- Available from the US Department of Labor poster office and regional offices or on the Internet at: http://freelaborlawposters.gov-docs.com/polygraph.html

Safety
- Occupational Safety and Health Act (OSHA) poster 2203 (Job Safety & Health Protection)

- Available from the U.S. Department of Labor poster office and regional offices or on the Internet at: http://198.234.41.214/w3/webpo2.nsf/pages/OnSitePoster Download
- OSHA also requires posting an annual summary of on-the-job injuries (OSHA Form 300A—Summary of Work-related Illnesses and Injuries)

Posters may be obtained from the government agency charged with enforcing a particular law. Most agencies have developed a single poster that satisfies the requirements of several different laws administered by that agency. Also, private companies publish posters that employers are required to post. Contact the following agencies to obtain these posters:

Equal Employment Opportunity Commission Office of Communication
1801 L Street, NW
Washington, DC 20507
(800) 435-7232 or (800) 669-3362

U.S. Department of Labor Posters
200 Constitution Avenue, NW, Room S-3502
Washington, DC 20210
(866) 4-USA-DOL

WORKERS' COMPENSATION

Physicians may think of Workers' Compensation in regard to the medical care it provides to other employers' workers. However, the physician-employer must cover his or her own employees with Workers' Compensation insurance.

Information that outlines your responsibilities can be obtained by contacting the Workers' Compensation Board in your state. An insurance agent is also a good resource for information about Workers' Compensation requirements.

OSHA WORKPLACE REQUIREMENTS

The Occupational Safety and Health Administration (OSHA) was enacted in 1970 to assure safe, healthful working conditions for employees. Employers are required to furnish employees with a place of employment that is safe from recognized hazards. In the medical office, bloodborne pathogens are the hazard of greatest concern.

It is the responsibility of every medical employer to obtain complete information for compliance with OSHA regulations. The *OSHA Handbook for Small Businesses*, which includes self-inspection checklists, is available from local OSHA offices.

HIRING EMPLOYEES

All employees need guidelines and rules to understand what is expected of them. A well-written job description is the best way of communicating a description of the duties for which an employee is responsible.

Your first priority should be to hire an experienced office manager. Expect to pay a higher wage to an experienced person, but by doing so you will recoup this extra expenditure in efficiency and dollars collected. Once the front office person has been hired, he or she can develop job descriptions and screen applicants for the clinical assistant and other staff, as needed.

Give a great deal of thought to the duties of the office manager and prepare a job description before beginning the advertising or hiring process. A job description usually includes the following elements:

Job Title	Name of the job.
Job Summary	A one- or two-sentence summary that defines the overall function of the job.
Job Qualifications	A brief listing of educational and experience qualifications.
Duties and Responsibilities	A list of the major job tasks describing what is to be accomplished.

Sample job descriptions for an office manager and a clinical assistant are provided at the end of this chapter.

Setting a Salary Range

Personnel salaries and benefits will be your largest single expense. You will want to hire the person with the best skills at the most affordable pay. Developing a salary range for each job title is the recommended way to set salaries. Staff salaries should be predicated on the following:

- How much the practice can afford to pay now and what you can probably pay next year.
- The average salary for the same job within the community for staff with the same level of experience and education.

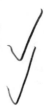

Before comparing salaries with other offices, make sure the job description is compared as well.

Sources for Developing a Pool of Candidates

The following are sources for developing a pool of candidates for a position at the practice:

- Office Managers' Professional Associations
- Community Colleges
- Private Vocational Schools
- Local Chapters of Health Care Organizations, such as the American Association for Medical Assistants, Medical Group Management Association, etc.
- Medical Societies' Placement Service
- Pharmaceutical Representatives
- Hospital Personnel Department
- Employment Agencies

Placing an Effective Classified Advertisement

The Civil Rights Act of 1964 (Title VII) also applies to the advertising, application, and hiring process. Ads must be carefully written to avoid any appearance of discrimination based on sex, age, race, religion, national origin, or disability. Use the basic components of the job description to write the ad, focusing on what the job requires rather than the type of person that is preferred. For screening purposes, when placing a newspaper advertisement, have candidates send their written resumes to a box number rather than listing a telephone number or your office address.

Preparing for the Interview

Review the written resumes that were received and choose at least five candidates with the qualifications that are required. Give each of these resumes a priority rating. Screen the top five applicants by telephone first. It may be preferable to have all five candidates come in for a face-to-face interview, or the choices can be narrowed down to two or three candidates.

Be organized in the face-to-face interviews, having a prepared list of questions to ask each candidate. This will allow you to compare the candidates on the same basis. Give each interviewee a copy of the job description and have him or her complete an EEOC-approved application form. Using an EEOC form will assure that you are not violating any of the Title IV statutes. These forms are available through the American Medical Association Publications Department, office supply stores, and most mail order catalogs offering forms for the medical office.

Every employer develops a unique interviewing style. You may want to begin your interviews by telling the candidate a little about yourself or your specialty. Share with the candidate why that particular geographic area was chosen, where you went to school, and what your philosophy is about the practice of medicine. Next, the following topics could be addressed:

- Ask if the candidate has reviewed the job description and whether there are questions about the essential functions of the job.

- Ask about the applicant's experience with each task listed on the job description. Ask how he or she performs these tasks in the current position or in former jobs. Write the answers on a separate piece of paper. Do not write on the job description, application form, or resume to avoid any comments that may be perceived as discriminatory.

- Ask open-ended questions that require the applicant to provide information. Avoid questions that can be answered yes or no.

- Remain neutral in your responses. Do not show approval or disapproval.

- Watch for nonverbal clues that indicate tension or anxiety.

- Zero in on topics of interest to you and investigate further.

- Quickly review your objectives.

- Document key points.

- Let the candidate know what happens next.

Interviewing Questions

Use the following list of questions with each candidate, making notes on a separate piece of paper, not on the resume or application.

- What did you like best about your last (current) position? What did you like least about it?

- Which of your past positions did you find most satisfying? Why?

- How would your last (current) supervisor describe you? In what area would he or she say you need the most improvement?

- What is one of your most significant on-the-job accomplishments?

- What academic areas of study interest you the most? What, if any, helped prepare you for your field?

- What did you like best about your last supervisor? What did you like least?

- What change would you (or did you) make in the last office you worked in?

- Describe your experiences in collecting money for medical bills.

- Which of your skills do you think you could develop here?

Checking References

Reference checking is vitally important to the medical employer, especially since they are increasingly being held responsible for negligent hiring decisions. Unfortunately, previous employers are generally reluctant to convey information on employees. Using finesse and gentle persuasion, however, you can usually obtain the information you need to make a hiring decision. One physician will usually be willing to tell another about the performance or abilities of an employee due to the significance of the decision. Be sure to thank the person for their cooperation. The following are steps that can be taken to ensure a smooth hiring process:

- Request that each applicant provide you with two or three references, preferably a former employer or supervisor.
- Call the references instead of accepting letters of reference at face value.
- Ask to speak to the applicant's immediate supervisor.
- Ask if the applicant is eligible for rehiring.
- Listen for what they do not say.

Orientation or Trial Period

When hiring, inform the new employee that he or she will be subject to a 90-day orientation or trial to be used for orientation and training. During this period, monitor the employee's attitude, work habits, and capabilities, and assure that he or she is receiving the proper instructions.

The employee or employer may end the employment relationship at-will at any time during this initial period, with or without cause, and without advance notice. Employees will assume regular status upon satisfactory completion of the orientation period.

Although during the start-up of a medical practice, all policies are not likely to be in a handbook or manual yet, developing written policies should be addressed in the earlier stages. If these policies are in place on the first day, present the employee with a copy of the policies, taking time to explain the basic work rules and regulations, including:

- Compensation and benefits
- Payroll deductions
- Vacation schedules and sick leaves
- Safety and health

Ask the employee to read the policies and offer to answer any questions. Address any other issues, such as dress codes, overtime, etc. After reviewing the policies, the employee should sign an acknowledgment form, which should be placed in the personnel file.

Personnel Files

Every employee, including the physicians, should have a well-maintained personnel file for the documents listed below. The typical file should contain all government-mandated forms and employee benefit enrollment forms, as applicable:

- Resume
- Employment Application
- Reference Checklist
- W-4 Form
- State Income Tax Form, if applicable
- Form I-9

- Payroll Set-Up Information
- Health Insurance Enrollment Form
- Long-Term Disability Enrollment Form
- 401(k) Enrollment Form
- Flex Benefits Form
- Personnel Policies Acknowledgment Form (Disclaimer)
- Attendance Records
- Employment Letter
- Salary Change Information
- Performance Reviews
- Warning or Disciplinary Letters
- New Employee Checklist
- Training Checklist
- Confidentiality Pledge
- Contact List in Case of an Emergency

Personnel files should be kept in a locked cabinet, accessible only to the designated employee responsible for maintenance. Employees have the right to access their files at any time, in the presence of a designated employee.

Personnel files should be retained for three years following termination. Applications of persons not hired should be maintained for one year.

PERFORMANCE APPRAISALS AND SALARY REVIEWS

Each employee should have a performance appraisal every year, either at a designated time for annual reviews or on the anniversary of the employee's hire date. Following are pointers on conducting a successful performance review:

- **Use a preprinted form.** Give the employee a copy a week or two in advance and ask for a self-evaluation on performance.
- **Conduct performance reviews separately.** Do not conduct a salary review during performance reviews. By combining the two, employees will concentrate on dollars rather than performance.
- **Allow adequate time.** Give the review process enough time to address the necessary topics; avoid rushing through!
- **Choose a quiet location.** Conduct the appraisal in a confidential atmosphere.
- **Highlight needed improvements.** Set specific goals and time lines for improvement.
- **Get a signature.** Ask the employee to sign off on the form acknowledging that the review was conducted.
- **End review on a good note.** Close the discussion with a compliment.

Salary Reviews

As a matter of necessity, salary increases must be based on practice profits. When funds are available, salary increases should be based on merit. Based on an employee's performance, merit raises can be motivators in that they recognize special effort or provide an incentive to improve. Know who is contributing, what they add to the practice, and how much. Do not be afraid to make a distinction; this is the point of merit raises.

Make sure all employees understand how salary increases are calculated and how they are given. Explain the process in the employee handbook.

Counseling, Discipline, and Termination

Managing a staff requires counseling, discipline, and some eventual terminations. Make every effort to work with your employees so that they may give their best to their duties. Note and file in the personnel file any disciplinary discussions held with the employee, documenting what was said and the subsequent response. These records will substantiate the reasons for termination, if this action becomes necessary. Having proper documentation reduces your exposure to loss from claims brought by a disgruntled staff member.

Before beginning the termination process, keep the following points in mind:

- Often, potential grounds for dismissal are present at the time an employee is hired. Be sure to check all past references thoroughly and have an understanding of how the applicant got along with previous coworkers, supervisors, and patients.
- Employees must understand the terms of any probationary period. It is important that they know the grounds for dismissal; that no advance notice will be given; and that severance pay and unemployment benefits may not be extended. (Check your state statutes.)
- All policies governing grounds for dismissal, disciplinary procedures, grievance procedures, etc, must be clearly outlined in the employee handbook. Be sure that all standards are equally and impartially applied to all employees.
- Any decision to terminate should be the final step in a clearly documented and well-defined process. Make sure all alternatives have been exhausted first.

You may have a host of reasons for beginning the disciplinary process for an employee. The employee must be made aware of unsatisfactory performance or behavior and be given a chance to improve; after giving ample opportunity to no avail, the employee should be terminated without delay.

THE EMPLOYEE HANDBOOK

A key part of an employer's communication program is the employee handbook. It provides information on basic rules and policies that affect job conditions and should be issued to each employee upon employment. The following general information will help in determining what to include in a handbook.

Your staff needs to understand:

- What is expected of them and what they can expect of you
- Your policies on wages, working conditions, and benefits
- What services the practice provides to patients

The employee handbook should reflect the mission and philosophy of the physician. Handbooks protect the employer. Guesswork can be eliminated when either the employer or employee can refer to a written policy.

Handbooks give employees a sense of security. With all the rules and policies in one place, each person knows what is expected. When benefits are listed and explained, each person knows what is provided. Handbooks can also help motivate employees.

Handbook Format

Choose a size for the handbook that is easy to use. Typical sizes are 5" × 7" or 8" × 10", either loose-leaf or bound. Loose-leaf notebooks allow for replacement of pages when policies change. Some employers use both formats—a small bound handbook for employees, and a loose-leaf policy and procedures manual for managers. Both books should include an employee acknowledgment form.

Make the booklet attractive; put it together in such a way that employees will want to read it. Consider these suggestions for making the contents easy to read:

- Limit the use of words with three or more syllables
- Keep each sentence 20 words or less
- Limit discussion of subjects to one page
- Use drawing, charts, and cartoons where applicable
- Leave at least one-quarter of each page blank
- Limit the number of pages

Choose a writing style and be consistent throughout. Use gender-neutral terminology. A handbook should cover what employees need to know to get along on the job—the policies and procedures that employees will encounter almost every day. Avoid subjects that change frequently, such as a lengthy and detailed description of benefits plans.

Table 11-1 provides a sample table of contents that can be used as a checklist for deciding what to include in a handbook.

TABLE 11-1

Handbook Sample Table of Contents

Welcome Letter and Introduction
- Letter of Appreciation to Current Employees
- Letter of Welcome to New Employees
- Purpose of Handbook
- Background of Practice
  - Organization Chart
  - Physician(s)' Biographical Information
- Equal Employment Opportunity Statement
- Suggestion and Complaint Procedures

Employment Policies and Procedures
- Nature of Employment
- Probationary Period
- Employment Relations
- Supervisor's Responsibilities
- Employee's Role and Responsibilities
- Work Schedules
- Rest and Meal Periods
- Overtime Policy
- Attendance and Punctuality
- Time Cards
- Personnel Records
- Payday
- Payroll Deductions
- Performance and Salary Reviews
- Resignation/Termination
- Telephone Use

Benefits
- Holidays
- Vacations
- Hospital and Medical Insurance
- Life Insurance
- Pension and Profit-Sharing
- Training
- Educational Assistance Program
- Service Awards
- Workers' Compensation
- Sick Leave
- Disability Leave
- Personal Leave
- Bereavement Leave
- Jury Duty
- Witness Duty

Safety
- Safety Rules
- Emergency Procedures
- Personal Protective Equipment
- Reporting Accidents

Employee Conduct and Disciplinary Action
- Standards of Conduct

TABLE 11-1 *Continued*

Handbook Sample Table of Contents

■ Confidentiality Policy
■ Smoking Policy
■ Drug, Alcohol, and Substance Abuse Policy (including testing, if applicable)
■ Sexual and Other Forms of Impermissible Harassment
■ Security Inspections
■ Solicitation
■ Personal Appearance and Dress Code
■ Corrective Discipline Procedures
Summary and Acknowledgment
■ Disclaimer Statement

Employee handbooks vary considerably due to individual needs and circumstances; therefore, the amount of information provided varies. A medical practice may also consider publishing Occupational Safety and Health Administration (OSHA), Clinical Laboratories Improvement Act (CLIA), and other government-regulated guidelines in its handbook. For the overall purpose of a handbook, however, mentioning these rules in passing is appropriate, while covering them more extensively in other documentation (ie, Policy Manual). Regardless, be sure the practice's acknowledgment form covers all policies.

Sample Job Descriptions

Figures 11-1 and 11-2 are samples of job descriptions for positions that can be found in a medical practice. These job descriptions can

FIGURE 11-1

Job Description—Office Manager

Position:	Office Manager
Reports to:	Physician(s)
Job Summary:	Responsible for all medical office activities, including accounting and financial procedures. Supervise all office personnel.

Specific Requirements:

- Furnish physician, accountant with account aging each month
- Conduct regular staff meetings
- Responsible for accounts payable system
- Supervise, train all front office personnel
- Assist in creating, updating business administration policies
- Update office personnel policy manual as needed
- Maintain controls on accounts receivable system
- Prepare financial reports at end of month for physician, accountant
- Approve all Medicaid, Medicare, and other write-offs in consultation with physician
- Approve credits, refunds to patient accounts
- Arrange personnel schedules and vacations
- Responsible for all hiring and terminating of office personnel
- Conduct performance, salary reviews for office personnel

Job Qualifications:

BA or AA degree in Business Administration required. Previous medical office experience also required. Supervisory experience preferred. Knowledge of medicolegal principles and medical ethics is necessary.

FIGURE 11-2

Job Description—Medical Assistant, Clinical

Position:	Medical Assistant, Clinical
Reports to:	Office Manager

Job Summary: Assist physician with patient examination and treatment. Also responsible for patient histories, routine lab procedures, collection, and preparation of specimens for transport to lab.

Specific Requirements:

- Maintain general appearance, cleanliness of exam rooms
- Sterilize instruments, maintain diagnostic equipment
- Prepare, replenish supplies; maintain inventory
- Prepare, drape patients for examination
- Take patient histories, height, weight, temperature
- Give certain medications, injections under physician supervision
- Assist in collection of specimens; instruct patients regarding preparation for tests
- Record laboratory, x-ray, EKG data on patient charts
- Receive and organize the handling of medication samples
- Dispose of contaminated and disposable items
- Perform other tasks as requested by office manager or physician

Job Qualifications:

Graduate of medical assistant training course or nursing program. Previous clinical experience and knowledge of anatomy, physiology, and terminology also required. Medical office experience helpful.

be used for preparing specific descriptions for jobs in a practice. They can also be used for performance appraisals and employee counseling. As responsibilities change, revise the descriptions accordingly.

CONCLUSION

Starting a medical practice involves becoming an employer or, at a minimum, functioning as a supervisor of staff members. The physician in a medical practice has to be knowledgeable of a number of employment laws and skillful in hiring and managing staff members.

chapter 12

Developing Policies and Procedures

INTRODUCTION

Every medical practice should have written policies and procedures for the completion of each task in the practice. Preparing written policies is a good exercise in thinking through the processes and examining their validity and accuracy. A well-written Policies and Procedures Manual will provide a training and orientation guide for new employees, and serve as an ongoing reference for the office staff.

DEVELOPING A POLICIES AND PROCEDURES MANUAL

The Policies and Procedures Manual should be prepared with greater detail and bound separately from the Employee Handbook. Each employee should sign a form that will be maintained in the employee's personnel file acknowledging that the policies and procedures have been read.

The Policies and Procedures Manual should accomplish the following:

- Provide step-by-step guidelines for completion of each task in the office
- Identify key personnel to use as resources for each task
- Include samples of forms to be used
- List frequently called telephone numbers
- Advise about miscellaneous office matters (eg, location of keys, how to reorder forms)

Specific policies and instructions should address the following functions:

- Communicating hospital and surgery charges
- Purchasing protocols
- Office collections routine
- Releasing patient records prerequisites
- Billing policies and follow-up
- Registering a patient
- Setting up a patient's file
- Completing a superbill

- Scheduling patient appointments
- Closing and reconciling day's activities
- Cleaning laboratory equipment
- Performing an EKG
- Scheduling a laboratory test
- Handling laboratory results (eg, notifying the patient, physician's responsibilities)

The physician must assume responsibility for the preparation of the Policies and Procedures Manual in the early stages. How each policy or procedure will be carried out or conducted should be defined. After the initial office set-up phase, this task can be turned over to the administrative staff for updates and maintenance. Figure 12-1 is an example of an appointment scheduling policy. Use it as a format for writing a specific manual.

TYPES OF APPOINTMENT SCHEDULES

Inefficient patient scheduling can significantly impede the progress of your day. There are many effective methods from which to choose. Experiment with different appointment schedules to learn what works best for the practice.

- **Typical format.** One patient scheduled every 15 minutes, with an extra 15 minutes allowed for complete physicals or new patients.
- **Wave method.** Three patients scheduled to arrive on the hour and half hour, based on the concept that one patient will always be early, another on time, and the third 5 to 10 minutes late.
- **Need method.** Patients for follow-up visits or minor illnesses are scheduled back-to-back. New patients, procedures, or physicals are scheduled as the first and last patient each morning and each afternoon.
- **Open access.** Patients are seen on the day they call, with designated time slots for types of visits.

Whatever method is used, let the office staff know that it is imperative patients wait no longer than 15 minutes without the physician being made aware of the situation. The staff should also be responsible for keeping the patients informed of any delays. Patients usually do not mind waiting an extra few minutes if they are regularly updated and given the opportunity to reschedule.

Your own responsibility for maintaining a prompt appointment schedule cannot be overstated. Being kept waiting is still the number one complaint of most patients. Patient satisfaction is crucial in today's health care market, and being on time goes a long way toward achieving patient satisfaction.

Consider the pointers in Table 12-1 when addressing scheduling issues. These tips will improve access and increase efficiencies, benefiting you and your patients. Ensure that your staff has this information available to them through the Policies and Procedures Manual.

FIGURE 12-1

Sample Policy—Appointment Scheduling

ABC Medical Practice Policies and Procedures Manual

Appointment Scheduling

When the doctor is in the office and running more than _____ minutes late:

■ Explanation to patients already in reception area and those arriving:

Suggest opportunity to reschedule? ❑ Yes ❑ No

■ Call patients not yet at office? ❑ Yes ❑ No

Suggest opportunity to reschedule? ❑ Yes ❑ No

When the doctor is in the office and running more than _____ minutes late:

■ Explanation to patients already in reception area and those arriving:

Suggest opportunity to reschedule? ❑ Yes ❑ No

If doctor is delayed at hospital, ER, nursing home, or other location:

■ Explanation to patients already in reception area and those arriving:

Suggest opportunity to reschedule? ❑ Yes ❑ No

■ Call patients not yet at office? ❑ Yes ❑ No

Suggest opportunity to reschedule? ❑ Yes ❑ No

Patients calling to cancel appointments should be asked the following questions:

_____

_____

_____

Be sure to document in chart and appointment book.

Call patients on *early call-in* those scheduled later in the week who might like to come in earlier.

Instruction/statements to callers who have previously been a *no-show:*

_____

Instructions/statements to patients being *worked-in:*

_____

_____

Office policy on non-emergency *drop-ins:*

_____

_____

Policy for when more than one family member hopes to be seen in an appointment time reserved for just one:

_____

_____

Office policy for patients arriving more than _____ minutes late:

_____

_____

Office policy for patients arriving early:

_____

_____

Office policy to follow when pharmaceutical sales representatives arrive without an appointment:

_____

_____

©1993 AMA Financing & Practice Services. Inc.

TABLE 12-1

Ten Tips for Efficient Scheduling

1.	Arrange office hours to fit community needs. Consider seeing patients during evening hours two or three times a week or Saturday mornings.
2.	Use an appointment scheduler customized according to physician preferences. In a partnership or group, scheduling preferences may vary by physician. Provide for evening and weekend coverage and vacations.
3.	Establish an office policy for screening telephone calls. Be sure to set aside specific times for callbacks.
4.	When an emergency results in a delay, explain the situation to waiting patients; give them a choice of waiting or rescheduling. Contact patients that are not yet in the office.
5.	When a patient requests an appointment time that is already filled, offer at least two other times that are available. Chances are the patient will choose one of the other times that were offered.
6.	Identify more lengthy appointment types, and "high risk, no show" patients (ie, new patients) and send them written or oral reminders.
7.	If canceling an appointment is necessary, notify the patient as soon as possible.
8.	If the physician makes house calls or visits to other institutions, schedule these trips realistically so they do not conflict with office hours.
9.	Do not overcrowd the schedule. Allow two or three times during the day for catching up, work-ins, or emergencies.
10.	On slow days, consider keeping a stand-by list available of patients who can be called in on short notice in case of cancellation.

CONCLUSION

For a myriad of reasons, every practice must have policies and procedures in place for *how we do that here*. Some of the issues are efficiency, structure, and liability. Many of the ways your practice does things will change as the staff grows and the practice builds its patient base. Written policies and procedures are essential for training and holding the staff accountable for the delivery of quality patient care.

chapter 13

Billing and Reimbursement Protocols

INTRODUCTION

Getting paid for services that were rendered in the medical practice is the difference between whether you will be able to afford to practice medicine or not—and it's harder than one may think! When you are starting out, it can seem hard to believe that collecting payments from patients and third-party payers will be the bane of your existence. The purpose of this chapter is to help you establish a sound protocol for billing and reimbursement that will enable you to collect and to expedite payment to fund your practice. The difference in whether payment is collected or not boils down to setting up a financial policy for payment and collections and implementing a course of action for filing claims with insurance carriers. Essential to the process is having well-trained practice staff who can relate to the patients and work with the third-party payers to get the job done.

COLLECTING FROM PATIENTS

Collection begins at the time the patient calls for the appointment and the scheduler explains the practice's financial policy. A simple request for an address so that the patient can be sent a practice brochure that includes the payment policy, or informing the patient that copayments and deductibles are due at the time of service will establish expectations of payment. Make sure you have a designated person assigned the responsibility of requesting payment for services. Having the right person in this role is critical to the collections process. This individual must be pleasant, mature, and well-trained. Following these simple and practical guidelines will increase the probability of collecting payment at the time of service.

Use collection etiquette or "good manners" when collecting from a patient by remembering these pointers:

- Respect the patient's privacy
- Use eye contact
- Address the patient by name
- Ask *how*, not if, the patient would like to pay
- Be prepared to explain the services and charges

- Be prepared to offer payment options if the patient is unable to pay in full
- Do not confront the patient
- Do not humiliate or embarrass the patient
- Smile and say "Thank you!"

At the initial or return visit, routinely follow these steps:

- Address the patient by name
- Itemize the fees
- Ask for payment
- Provide payment options
- Remember to say "Thank you!"

If the patient has a previous balance or partial payment, approach the situation as follows:

- Use a polite, matter-of-fact attitude to approach a patient about a previous balance to maximize the opportunity to collect
- Address the patient by name
- Itemize the fees for today's visit

For more information on collecting from the patient, including preparation of your practice's financial policy, see the *Billing the Patient* section later in this chapter.

Collecting at the Time of Service

The best opportunity you have to collect your fee is to ask patients to pay while still in the office. Collect copayments, deductibles, and open balances either before or after the office visit by asking courteously, "How would you like to pay today? By cash, check, or credit card?" Speak matter-of-factly, using the patient's name. Be willing to explain the charges or answer any questions.

COLLECTING FROM THIRD-PARTY PAYERS

Much more challenging than collecting from your patients is the complexity of attaining reimbursement from insurers. The marketplace consists of a variety of plans and payers that include indemnity plans, discounted arrangements, and government-funded programs, such as Medicare, Medicaid, and workers' compensation programs. Some insurers have many plans that you will be obligated to adhere to if you are a participating provider. Whatever your specialty, you will face many obstacles and much resistance to reimbursement for services rendered.

Interfacing with Insurance Companies

From 80 to 90 percent of your patients are covered by some form of insurance. An efficient computer system will take most of the hassles out of claims processing, yet there are still obstacles to overcome in order to collect reimbursements. The more you know about how insurance companies work, the more successful you will be in collecting. Following is basic information on various plans and an overview of how they will affect your ability to collect your charges.

Indemnity Plans

The traditional insurance companies are known as indemnity or commercial insurance plans. Sometimes called 80/20 plans, their marketing materials typically state that they pay 80 percent of the patient's medical bill, and the patient only pays the remaining 20 percent after an annual deductible is met. This type of advertising is misleading to the patient, because these companies base the 80 percent they pay on what they term a usual and customary reimbursement (UCR). The insurance company's UCR for a particular service is seldom, if ever, the same as your fee for that same service. Insurance companies generally do not explain how they establish their usual and customary fees.

Example:

You charge a patient $1,000 for repair of an inguinal hernia. The indemnity insurance plan says the usual and customary fee is $800, so they pay 80 percent of $800, not 80 percent of $1,000. The patient then is responsible for paying $360 to the physician instead of the $200 (or 20 percent of $1,000) they expected to pay. Often, the patient receives an explanation of benefits (EOB) that includes a statement similar to this:

"Your physician's fee is higher than the usual and customary fee for this service/procedure. The usual and customary fee for this procedure is $800, so we are reimbursing 80 percent of $800."

Without an understanding of how the insurance company pays for a particular procedure, or how this fee is calculated, the patient is apt to be annoyed with the physician. Therefore, it is wise to conduct some patient education before performing a service or surgical procedure. Explain to the patient that the fee for the service may not be the same as the insurance company's reimbursement. Also explain that your fees are set so that you can provide a high-quality service, pay your expenses, and remain competitive in the marketplace. Open communications are what keep patients happy and set successful physicians apart from their peers.

Managed Care Plans

New physicians entering the marketplace have an advantage in that they grew up with the managed care concept. Physicians that have been in private practice for many years have had to learn a new payment process and modify the way they view patient care.

Several types of plans are offered in most areas, and most insurers sell some type of managed care plans that generally pay the provider on a discounted fee for service or a capitated basis.

Discounted Fee-for-Service Plans

In a discounted fee-for-service plan, the payer/insurance plan negotiates with the physician for a discount off the regular fee for a particular service in exchange for the promise of a potential increase in patients. Generally, the physician receives no guarantee in the number of patients he or she will receive from the plan. These plans are typically called Preferred Provider Organizations (PPO), Point of Service Plans (POS), or Health Maintenance Organizations (HMO).

Capitated Plans

In a capitated arrangement, the physician agrees to provide a specified list of services to each patient assigned to the practice for a set dollar amount each month (ie, per member per month). The insurer pays the physician this specified amount whether or not the physician sees the patient in the office. The amount may range from $3 per patient to $15 per patient depending on the specialty and the services that the physician is required to provide within the capitated amount. This is often termed a risk-sharing arrangement.

Example:

The physician has 100 patients assigned to his or her practice for which the insurer pays a capitated fee of $15 per member/per month (pm/pm), or a total of $1,500. If the physician sees 20 of these patients in a month and these patients require a total of $1,800 worth of services, she has lost $300. However, if the physician sees only 5 of the 100 patients in a month and their services total $200, she has made a gross profit of $1,300. Seeing the risk involved in this arrangement is easy.

This example is an oversimplification of how reimbursement works in a managed care market. It is intended to explain the various types of insurance plans that you will encounter in a private practice. Before accepting and/or signing any kind of agreement with a managed care organization, the practice should understand the complexities of the system. Also, have an attorney or experienced health care consultant review any contract before signing it.

Workers' Compensation Insurance

All employers must provide workers' compensation insurance to cover the medical and disability expenses incurred by the worker from a job-related injury. Many states administer Workers' Compensation Insurance billing directly. In these states, the physician sends the claims directly to the state's agency. Other states require employers to contract with an insurance company for payment of work-related claims. In either case, benefits and payments are predetermined by legislation, based upon the state and the company. Request a packet of information from your State Workers' Compensation Board in preparation for accepting patients with work-related injuries and before processing claims.

When accepting a patient for a work-related injury, follow these guidelines in order to receive reimbursement for your services:

■ Before seeing the patient, get authorization for treatment from the employer.

- Try to get a written request for treatment from the employer.

- If a written request is not possible, call the employer for authorization. Use a simple *Telephone Consent* form to record the authorization.

- The employer must notify the insurance company of the injury. Without a *first report of injury*, reimbursement will be delayed.

- Treat Workers' Compensation claims as any insurance claim, filed in the unpaid claim file, and routinely followed up.

- The first claim form should reach the insurance company within 10 days of first treatment, even if treatment is completed.

- Physicians cannot bill patients for treatment of work-related injuries.

Insurance Filing and Follow-Up

Insurance claims processing consumes a large portion of administrative time. Setting up workable policies and systems initially will help assure that insurance reimbursement provides a steady flow of cash into the practice.

Most medical management software can print the HCFA 1500 insurance form used for filing a claim with Medicare and Medicaid. This form is used, as well, with indemnity insurance carriers and managed care plans. Automation simplifies the filing process and allows the practice to submit claims daily, if desired. However, the claim filing process is only one small part of the reimbursement process. Monitoring the filed claims and assuring that insurers are paying them quickly requires much more effort.

Develop a claim filing protocol similar to the following example to streamline this process:

- File claims at least twice weekly; daily is preferable.

- Check all claims for accuracy and completeness of information before mailing. Most insurance companies promise a 30-day turnaround time for payments if they receive a clean claim. Some states have enacted legislation requiring payers to pay claims within a certain time frame. Be aware of the laws in your state and report any violations to the proper authorities.

- Print out a Claims Pending Report daily; call the insurance carrier on all claims that they have not paid within 30 days of the filing date. If your computer cannot generate this report, enter filed claims on an insurance log. Enter the date, the patient's name, the insurance company, and the amount filed on the log sheet. Check the log sheets every day to determine which claims have not been paid in 30 days and follow-up by telephone.

- Call the insurance companies to ask about an unpaid claim. Calling is more effective than simply resubmitting the claim. If the insurance company says it has not received the claim, then it must be resubmitted.

- Print out an aged accounts analysis *by payer* each month to learn which companies pay on time and which ones habitually exceed a 30-day turnaround time. (This is not a standard report on every system. It is worthwhile to request that the system be set up to provide this report.)
- Call the plan administrator and request an explanation of the plan's poor payment habits. Most managed care contracts guarantee a 30-day reimbursement schedule if the claims are submitted in order. If you do not receive your payments as agreed, it may be a sign that the plan is in financial trouble. If the payment problems persist, you may wish to terminate the contract.
- Make contractual adjustments at the time they make the payment.
- Conduct a periodic review of Explanation of Benefits (EOBs). An EOB statement, similar to a check stub, accompanies every insurance payment. Compare the EOB with the filed claim to assure that the insurer is paying claims appropriately, without reductions or denials.

Consistent follow-up is the key to satisfactory reimbursement. If insurance claims are produced on a file-and-forget method, you may find yourself with a cash flow shortfall. Give employees a copy of the written policy. Make them accountable for following these routines.

BILLING THE PATIENT

Patients are personally responsible to you, the physician, for the payment of medical services that were rendered, even if they have insurance. You are not obligated to file the patient's insurance claims unless you have a contract with the insurance company. These contracted agreements include Medicare, Medicaid, and Managed Care Plans. Agreeing to file a patient's insurance and wait for the reimbursement is a service you provide to your patients. This service is important, and it is one that most practices provide. However, make sure your patients understand that payment is ultimately their responsibility.

Establish a written financial policy that you can present to your patients before they receive treatment. This financial policy should explain payment expectations and your policy on filing insurance claims. The following is a list of important points to include in the written financial policy:

- A statement that payment for services is expected at the time of service unless arrangements are made prior to treatment.
- The office will file insurance claims for services rendered, but the patients are not relieved of responsibility for payment because they have insurance.
- Patients must pay copays or deductibles due before surgical procedures are performed and at the time services are rendered.

- Statements are mailed every 30 days. Any balance left unpaid after 90 days will be turned over to a collection agency.
- Financial arrangements can be made for payment of bills that are more than $XXX (you choose your limit).

Statements sent to patients should itemize the procedures and include the entire amount due, even if an insurance company will pay most of it. Many practice management software programs will produce statements that show both the amount presumed covered by insurance and the portion for which the patient is responsible.

Patients should receive statements regularly for any outstanding amount. Your billing cycle can be set up in several ways. The traditional method is to send all statements at the end of each month. Other methods include sending statements twice monthly, one half on the 15th and one half on the 30th. The third method is to send some statements out each week according to letters of the alphabet. These last two billing methods spread the cash flow and the associated payment posting work more evenly throughout the month.

The following are a few billing tips for the practice:

- Send each patient a billing statement within 30 days after the date of service.
- Call each patient who has an unpaid bill 45 days after the date of treatment. Ask if a problem has prevented payment of the bill. Make notes of any comments made by the patient.
- If the patient says that he or she cannot pay the full amount of the bill, offer to set up a payment schedule.
- Remind the patient of a previous balance.
- If the patient makes a partial payment, set up (and record) a payment agreement.
- Offer the patient a payment envelope.
- Remember to say "Thank you!"

Officially terminating the patient/physician relationship is important when they do not meet financial obligations. The physician cannot refuse to treat an established patient who owes the practice money unless the relationship has been formally terminated. See Chapter 14, *Loss Prevention and Risk Management,* for more information on patient termination.

As with insurance filing and billing, a structured process for patient billing and follow-up is the most important factor in achieving reimbursement. Table 13-1 offers a sample of a patient billing and follow-up schedule.

USING A COLLECTION AGENCY

Approximately 2 percent of patients do not pay their medical bills. After you have exhausted all your in-house collection techniques, it may be best to turn some accounts over to a collection agency.

TABLE 13-1

Patient Billing and Follow-up Schedule

Action	Time Frame
Send 1st statement	Within 30 days of date of service
Send 2nd statement	30 days after date of service
Call patient with unpaid bill; if patient says unable to pay, set up payment schedule	45th day after treatment date
Call patient; record comments	75th day after date of service
Send 3rd statement	90th day after date of service
Send letter stating that payment is due within 20 days or account will be turned over for collection	100th day

Choose a collection agency carefully, being mindful that the agency's collection methods reflect on your practice. Talk with other physicians or office managers to see which agency they are using. Ask if they are satisfied with the services they receive and what percentage of accounts turned over for collection are paid. Collection agencies typically show a collection success rate of less than 25 percent. Use the checklist in Figure 13-1 on the next page for selecting a credible collection agency.

Besides the items listed above, the following points should be considered:

- Get copies of all the letters the agency will send to your patients.
- Do not turn over accounts of less than $50.
- Make a note on the patient's ledger card that you have turned over the account.
- Never pay commission up front.
- Make sure accounts can be recalled any time.
- Have a written agreement. Read the fine print.
- Do not allow the agency to litigate an account without your permission.
- Report changes in the collection status of an account to the agency.
- Keep a log of all accounts in collection. Enter the name, date turned over, amount due, amount the patient paid, and the net back.
- Use two agencies simultaneously so their efficiency can be evaluated.
- Establish a time limit on how long an agency is entitled to a percentage of amounts collected after an account is withdrawn.

USING CREDIT CARDS TO ENHANCE COLLECTIONS

Acceptance of credit cards for payment of medical bills is routine in most offices. This offers an excellent option for physicians because it brings funds into the practice immediately, and transfers the risk of nonpayment to the credit card companies.

FIGURE 13-1

Checklist for Selecting a Collection Agency

Question	Answer
1. Is the agency a member of the American Collectors Association?	
2. Is the agency in total compliance with the Fair Debt Collection Practices Act?	
3. What percentage of their business is medical?	
4. How are the accounts broken down per collector?	
5. How many accounts per collector?	
6. Does the agency have a training program?	
7. Does the monthly collection summary show when they listed the account and how much was paid?	
8. What are the agency's hours?	
9. Will they work accounts between 6:00 p.m. and 9:00 p.m. when most patients are available?	
10. How quickly does the account get on the desk of a collector?	
11. What reports do they provide?	
12. Does the agency report non-payers to the Credit Bureau?	
13. How long will the agency work on an account before they deem it noncollectible?	
14. How much commission do they charge?	

Almost every bank offers vendor/merchant accounts that will allow you to deposit your credit card payments into the bank for processing. Some credit card companies will transfer the funds to your bank electronically so that you have access to the money immediately.

Each bank sets its own service charge for processing credit card transactions that are generally based on a percentage of your overall deposits and range from 2 to 8 percent. The service charge is often negotiable. If you have no deposit history with the bank, your negotiating clout may not be very strong. If the bank accepts electronic transfers of your funds from the credit card companies, the service charge should be lower.

Your credit card merchant account does not have to be in the same bank as your checking account. However, you will find that it is more convenient, and you will generally receive favorable service charge rates from your own bank.

This is the process for establishing a credit card account:

■ Visit the bank where you have your office account and inquire about setting up a merchant account for the acceptance of credit card deposits. Ask the rate of their service charges. (Do not accept their first offer; attempt to negotiate the lowest rate possible.)

■ Once an account has been established, you will be assigned a merchant number. The bank will typically provide all necessary materials for accepting credit cards such as charge slips, credit slips, deposit slips, electronic card reader, etc. They will also provide you with the machine that allows you to obtain approval from the credit card companies and have the funds electronically transferred into its account. This process may vary; every bank's credit card department has established protocols for merchant accounts.

■ Ask the bank representative if having a bank employee come to your office is possible to set up the electronic transmittal unit and explain to your staff how the credit card process works.

Controlling the accounts receivable process will assure that your practice is financially successful. Collecting monies due is not a process that runs on its own. The physician should take an interest in this process. Establish measurable goals and make employees accountable for responsibilities in the process.

WRITING A COLLECTION POLICY FOR YOUR PRACTICE

During the early stages of a practice start-up—before bad habits have a chance to develop—institute a collection policy. Table 13-2 is an example of policies and procedures that have been set up for handling collections at a practice.

TABLE 13-2

Policies and Procedures for Handling Collections

COLLECTIONS POLICY

Policy

Practice staff charged with collection of receivables will operate within established legal guidelines and protocols during the pursuit of payment on outstanding patient account balances.

Purpose

To define guidelines for collection of patient account balances.

Procedure

■ Practice staff members DO NOT engage in any conduct that may be construed as harassment, oppression, or abuse of anyone in connection with collection of debt. Conduct disallowed includes, but is not limited to:
- verbal abuse
- threats to inform debtor's employer of debt
- disclosure of debt to any third party
- invasion of individual's privacy.

■ Telephone collections may occur Monday through Friday, 8:00 AM to 9:00 PM, Saturday, 8:00 AM to 5:00 PM, unless instructed otherwise by the patient.

■ Patients may be contacted at their place of employment, unless otherwise instructed by the patient.

■ All accounts must be approved by the physician or practice administrator before referral to a collection agency.

■ Threats of legal action may not be used UNLESS such action is likely.

ACCOUNT RESPONSIBILITIES/STANDARDS

Policy

The office staff must pursue collection of outstanding patient account balances and perform all subsequent write-offs without delay.

Purpose

To expedite reimbursements on patient accounts and to reduce outstanding accounts receivable.

Procedure

■ Maintain the standard or better.
■ Review Explanation of Benefits (EOBs) daily and pursue unpaid services.
■ Report trends regarding changes or delays in reimbursement from payers to Manager.
■ Prepare timely write-offs, taking adjustments at the time of posting.
■ Take bad debt write-offs as soon as an account is determined to be noncollectible.

Recommendations

Use the collection feature on the practice management system to facilitate timely follow-up, or use a tickler system to remind you.

TABLE 13-2 *Continued*

Policies and Procedures for Handling Collections

ACCOUNT FOLLOW-UP

Policy

Manager assigns accounts to the appropriate practice staff for timely follow-up and account maintenance.

Purpose

To ensure all patient accounts receive timely follow-up and subsequent account maintenance.

Procedure

■ All accounts over 30 days old are reviewed and pursued for prompt payment, which is accomplished by following up with the insurance companies.

■ The tickler system or the practice management system should be used to systematically follow up on accounts. (NOTE: A manual tickler system can simply consist of writing the patient's account number on a designated calendar date to make the return status call.)

■ All follow-up calls should be documented in the practice management system, noting the following information:

 - Name and telephone number of the insurance company that was contacted

 - Name of contact person at the insurance company

 - Brief summary of discussion

 - Date payment is expected

PROBLEM PAYERS

Policy

Accounts receivable issues should be identified and resolved in a timely manner. Problematic issues are documented and should be followed up by management.

Purpose

To ensure all contracted payers are compliant with specific contract terms and that all noncontract payers remit appropriate reimbursement in a timely manner.

Procedure

■ Notify physician or manager of any problem-related issues involving payers.

■ Attempt to quantify the scope of the problem (ie, total claims outstanding, the dollar and aging associated with those claims).

■ Once the information is quantified, contact the payer's provider representative to discuss resolution of the issue within 15 days. The conversation should be documented and a letter sent to the provider representative confirming the conversation and the expected outcome.

■ If no resolution is reached by the 16th business day, contact the provider representative to inform of the intent to send a certified letter to the medical director requesting resolution within 15 days.

■ A copy of this letter should also be sent to the patient's employer group, attention benefits manager.

■ If resolution has not been received within the stipulated 15 days, the next option will be to consider engaging legal representation or a health care consultant to resolve the issue.

Recommendations

Thoroughly review the payer contracts for all restrictions and stipulations. Before entering into any contract with a payer, have a legal representative or consultant review the agreement.

CONCLUSION

In addition to delivering high-quality patient care and service, do a good job collecting from patients and third-party payers and your practice will be on the road to success. Have good billing and collection protocols in place and a well-trained staff to carry them out. Get help from an experienced health care consultant to help the practice get off to a good start.

chapter 14

Loss Prevention
and Risk Management

INTRODUCTION

Risk management is the core of successful practice management. The practice must prioritize its risk plan and create operational consistency. Without a good risk management program, you may pay some grave consequences, such as being removed from the Medicare program, being hit with fraud and abuse charges, or facing noncompliance with other government regulations.

Risk management has evolved beyond reducing exposure to professional liability actions to more complex issues. Now, risk management has grown to protecting the practice's financial and physical assets through insurance and proper management techniques and behaviors. A good risk management program will reduce practice expenses and limit exposure.

Risk management is more than a program to prevent lawsuits: it is how a medical practice provides care for patients and improves the quality of life for physicians and their staff. Successful risk management requires close attention to building strong physician-patient relationships and capable physician-administrator teams.

CRITICAL TASKS IN RISK MANAGEMENT

Following are the critical tasks involved in risk management:

1. **Maintain legal compliance with corporate structure.** As presented in Chapter 2, *Choosing an Organizational Structure,* business entities (ie, sole proprietorships, partnerships, corporations, Sub S corporations) have specific requirements for governance and tax reporting. Once the business entity is established, make sure that you maintain compliance with the legal and tax guidelines applicable to your organization. Seek professional advice and assistance from your attorney and accountant.

2. **Develop record-keeping procedures.** Maintain records for your practice in relationship to your organizational structure. If yours is a corporation or partnership, you must live by your bylaws and articles of incorporation or by the decisions of the partners. Your attorney and accountant can advise you on record-keeping requirements.

3. **Develop conflict resolution and grievance procedures.**
    Managing risk encompasses personnel management,
    operational policies and procedures, OSHA compliance,
    and labor laws. The ability to resolve internal and external
    conflicts is important. Set up the necessary processes to
    anticipate, address, and resolve problems before they become
    issues that put your practice at risk of a lawsuit, fines,
    or penalties.

4. **Obtain liability insurance.** Liability protection includes
    professional malpractice, directors' and officers' (for
    corporations), errors and omissions, medical, disability, and
    property insurances for your employees, business, and
    property. Before purchasing such insurances, assess the level of
    risk. Seek the advice of a reputable and trustworthy insurance
    agent or broker.

5. **Establish personnel and property security plans.** Establish
    a policy for unauthorized or inappropriate use of the Internet
    and electronic equipment and resources, such as computers,
    telephones, and other technology that are available to practice
    staff. These policies and protections should be a part of your
    employee handbook and administered consistently.

6. **Develop and implement quality assurance and patient
    satisfaction programs.** Following are examples of a loss
    prevention program to promote quality and satisfaction:
    –   Identify existing or potential patient care problems
    –   Establish criteria for patient care responsibility
    –   Measure and monitor the actual performance of the staff
    –   Investigate and resolve problems or complaints
    –   Monitor the corrective action
    –   Educate employees about government regulatory programs
        and the record-keeping requirements for each program
    –   Provide continuing education for both employees and
        patients

7. **Establish confidentiality policies.** Protect your practice by
    having employees sign confidentiality agreements from the
    employee handbook stating that violations of practice
    confidentiality and breaching patient confidentiality will be
    cause for termination. Medical records must also be protected as
    a part of the practice's policies and procedures. The policy must
    address federal, state, and local regulations surrounding privacy
    and confidentiality, medical records policy and distribution, and
    organizational information flow.

8. **Negotiate and comply with contractual arrangements.** The
    practice is responsible for negotiating contracts, performing due
    diligence on them, and understanding them. If you are unable
    to get enough information on the company or understand the
    contract language or its implications, seek outside assistance
    from a third party, such as a reputable consulting firm.

9. **Maintain compliance with government mandates.** Many laws
    result in somewhat nebulous policies and procedures, such as
    self-referrals and safe harbors. Thorough knowledge of federal,

state, and local laws and regulations regarding human resources, OSHA, self-referral, fraud and abuse, Medicare fraud and abuse, ADA, anti-trust, and research is mandatory—regardless of the vagueness of their interpretations.

10. **Develop a network of advisors.** Seek advice and assistance from trusted professionals (eg, accountants, lawyers, insurance companies, coding experts, local Medicare office, consultants) for knowledge about the rules and changes that are continually occurring.

ADDRESSING AREAS OF RISK THROUGH OPERATIONAL IMPROVEMENTS

The following sections individually address each area of practice operation and provide suggestions for developing a loss prevention protocol in these areas.

Scheduling

A common source of patient dissatisfaction and subsequent increase in the risk of a professional liability claim is the length of time the patient must wait for an appointment with the physician. The busy practice staff may not realize that when a patient endures long waits, they perceive a lack of concern. Consider these details when scheduling patients:

- The length of time it takes to get an appointment
- The receptionist's demeanor
- Whether the receptionist asks patients who call for an appointment permission before putting them on hold
- The average length of time a patient is left on hold on the telephone

Patients become annoyed if the wait time exceeds 15 minutes. The maximum time a patient should wait in the reception area is 30 minutes. Any longer than 30 minutes and the patient becomes dissatisfied. To decrease the patient's wait time, follow these recommendations:

- Schedule extra time for new patients or special procedures.
- Allow enough time before and after seeing patients. Avoid over-booking patients.
- Inform patients of any delays in the appointment schedule and the cause for the delay.
- Call patients at home to advise of any expected delays.
- Block time each day for walk-ins and emergencies. Fill these times no earlier than the evening before.

Additional pointers on scheduling are introduced in Chapter 12, *Developing Policies and Procedures.*

Documentation of appointment information is almost as critical as the progress note itself in relation to managing risk. Always track all appointment questions and concerns using the following guidelines:

- Record missed or canceled appointments in the patient's chart.
- Do not erase, white out, or otherwise obliterate any appointment in the appointment book or computer schedule.
- Document any attempts to reach the patient to reschedule a missed appointment. If the patient's condition warrants, send a certified letter.

(See also Chapter 12, *Developing Policies and Procedures*.)

Billing and Collections

Many malpractice claims are a response to collection efforts that are offensive. A written collection policy assures that all practice staff members know what the policy is and how to handle each billing and collection situation (see Table 13-2, *Policies and Procedures for Handling Collections*, in Chapter 13, *Billing and Reimbursement Protocols*). In addition, also consider addressing the following issues in the policy as a measure of risk management:

- Patient education—letting the patient know before the first appointment about fees and payment requirements.
- A review procedure for circumstances that require special action.
- The patient's past payment history.
- The quality of care.
- The patient's satisfaction. If the patient balks at paying a bill, discuss it to reach an agreeable payment arrangement, if possible.
- The cost of legal action versus how much money the patient owes. Obtain information from the appropriate small claims court in the area.
- Having the physician review every chart before initiating aggressive collection procedures.
- Understanding of patients' rights concerning privacy and the physician-patient relationship. (Do not send any medical information to a collection agency.)
- Awareness of Fair Debt Collection Act. (Periodically evaluate the collection agency's practices.)

(See also Chapter 13, *Billing and Reimbursement Protocols*.)

Environment

The patient develops a first impression of the kind of medical care that will be provided from the practice environment. If the surroundings are pleasant, clean, and convenient, patients will more likely view you as competent and providing quality care. Consider the following suggestions as a part of your risk management plan:

- To prevent patient injury, evaluate the facility to ensure easy access. Check all patient care areas, including the parking lot, to identify potential safety hazards.
- Provide comfortable office furnishings to allow the patient to feel at ease. Check furnishings periodically to assure that they are in good condition. Take steps to ensure cleanliness and good housekeeping. Messy or dirty offices create a negative

impression and significantly affect the patient's perception of quality of care.

■ Have furnishings that meet the needs of various patients. Soft and/or low seating is problematic for women who are pregnant, senior citizens, and persons with disabilities. Remove obstacles that could cause tripping or falls. Breakable and small objects can be hazardous to children.

■ Keep the room at a comfortable temperature and provide plenty of lighting.

Medical Equipment

Patients are often injured because of faulty or improper use of equipment. The practice administrator should institute a policy of regular maintenance and use of all equipment, in addition to the following training practices:

■ Train all employees on the proper use of equipment.

■ Document the training, time, and place in each employee's personnel file.

■ Calibrate all equipment as recommended by the manufacturer.

■ Maintain a log of all equipment maintenance and service.

■ Report to the malpractice insurance carrier any patient injury associated with a piece of equipment. Remove the equipment and all its collateral equipment from service.

■ Avoid tampering with the equipment or sending it to the manufacturer for repair until the insurance company has been notified and they offer instructions.

■ **Do not document any assumptions about an equipment malfunction or improper usage in the medical record.**

Emergencies

Your risk management plan should also include a written protocol for handling a medical emergency, such as the following:

■ Post emergency numbers, such as ambulances, hospitals, poison control, etc, next to all telephones.

■ Require all staff to stay current on cardiopulmonary resuscitation (CPR).

■ If the office has emergency equipment and/or medications, train all staff to use such equipment and drugs. Not having this equipment on hand is better than to have untrained employees using it. There is often less liability in doing nothing than in doing something incorrectly.

■ Conduct periodic emergency drills to role-play various emergency scenarios.

Confidentiality

Communication between the patient and physician is confidential and critical to the patient-physician relationship. The patient's right to confidentiality extends to all members of the practice staff. Many suits are filed based on breach of confidential information. Only the patient has the right to decide what information may be revealed to others.

A risk management plan will institute the following constraints for the practice staff:

- All personal data, medical notes, and billing information are confidential and may not be communicated to anyone without the patient's written consent.

- Do not discuss a patient's illness with any staff member who does not need to know.

- Do not discuss a patient's illness with family members or friends except in the presence of and with the consent of the patient.

- Loose talk that is overheard by others can be the basis for a defamation or invasion of privacy suit. Watch your voice volume; and pay attention to who is nearby.

- Conduct a confidentiality audit of your office. Test to see how easy it is to overhear conversations. If necessary, install some soundproofing or white noise measures.

- Avoid discussing a patient's medical care on a cellular telephone with either the patient or anyone else. Sometimes police scanners and radios intercept cellular telephone conversations.

Handling Patient Complaints

A patient shows dissatisfaction and intentions to sue long before the legal papers are served. A staff member may be the first to be aware of a patient complaint. All complaints must be brought to the physician's attention, no matter how minor the incident may seem. No complaint should be ignored. The risk management plan should include the following guidelines:

- Institute a formal complaint policy in the office. Use an incident report form and a complaint log to track the occurrence and disposition of all patient complaints. Do not enter this information in the patient's medical record.

- Notify the physician of the complaint on the day it is received.

- Respond to the complaint quickly and follow up with the patient.

Termination of the Patient-Physician Relationship

The inferred contract between a patient and physician begins not when they make an appointment, but when examination or treatment begins. Once a patient-physician relationship has been established, the physician is not free to terminate the relationship without formal, written notification. The patient-physician relationship continues until it is ended by one of the following circumstances:

- The patient has no need of further care.
- The patient terminates the relationship.
- The physician formally terminates the relationship.

Failure to terminate may constitute patient abandonment and bring about fines or legal action if the patient is harmed by the abandonment.

There may be circumstances in which it is deemed necessary to terminate the patient-physician relationship. For example, perhaps the patient is noncompliant, and it is believed that continued treatment would increase the chances of a complication or poor outcome. Maybe the patient is rude or abusive, or maybe the physician and the patient just do not get along. Or, perhaps the patient routinely fails to pay his or her bills. Any of these reasons and many others may be a basis to terminate a patient from the practice. A physician, however, **cannot** refuse to give a patient an appointment because the patient has not paid the bill without first terminating the patient-physician relationship. Terminating the patient-physician relationship can be accomplished by sending the patient a **certified, return receipt letter.**

Once the patient is released, be sure to follow some specific guidelines to minimize the chance of being sued for abandonment. Observe the following principles as a matter of your risk management strategy:

- First, put the notice in writing. The reason may or may not be stated, but can be one of the following:
  - If for noncompliance, say so clearly in the letter.
  - If for personality conflict, an unpaid bill, or for a reason not to be made public, avoid stating the reason in writing.
- Send the letter by certified mail, return receipt requested. Keep the receipt in the patient's file, along with a copy of the letter. (See Figure 14-1 for a sample of a Patient Discharge Letter.)

The amount of time a physician is required to give a patient to seek alternative health care varies in each state. Contact your local medical society or seek counsel from an attorney to find the answer. This termination process protects you from having to see the patient who fails to follow your suggested treatment plan.

The patient-physician relationship is the foundation of medical law. Upon it rests the legal rights and obligations of both patients and physicians.

Rights of the Patient

The physician and staff members must be aware of certain legal rights that belong to the patient. They are as follows:

- The right to choose the physician from whom to receive treatment.

F I G U R E 14-1

Sample Discharge Letter

JAMES L. SMITH, MD
100 North Main Street
Anytown, USA

Telephone: (202) 555-1212
(Certified Mail-Return Receipt Requested)

[NAME]
[Address]
[City, State, Zip]

Dear _____:

I find it necessary to inform you that I am withdrawing from further professional attendance upon you for the reason that you have persisted in refusing to follow my medical advice and treatment.

Since your condition requires medical attention, I suggest that you place yourself under the care of another physician without delay. If you so desire, I will be available to attend you for a reasonable time after you have received this letter, but in no event for more than 30 days.

This should give you ample time to select a physician of your choice from the many competent practitioners in this city. With your approval, I will make available to this physician your case history and information regarding the diagnosis and treatment that you have received from me.

Very truly yours,

_____, MD

- The right to say whether medical treatment will begin and to set limits on the care provided.
- The right to know before the treatment begins:
  - what it will consist of
  - what effect it will have on the body
  - what are the inherent dangers
  - what it will cost

Consent to Treatment

Legal consequences for treating a patient without properly informed consent include charges of assault and battery and negligence. For emphasis, take note of the following:

- Treating a patient without permission is grounds for an assault and battery charge
- Treating a patient with the patient's consent, but failing to explain the inherent risks of a procedure, could result in a charge of negligence

Implied consent is reflected in the patient's actions, such as having a prescription filled or accepting an injection.

Expressed consent is an oral or written acceptance of the treatment. Obtain the written form of expressed consent when the proposed treatment involves surgery, experimental drugs or procedures, or high-risk diagnostic or treatment procedures.

Informed Consent to Treatment

The fiduciary relationship between the physician and the patient is based upon trust and confidence. The nature of this relationship obligates the physician to act for the benefit of the patient. Contained in this obligation is the physician's duty to voluntarily inform the patient of all relevant information concerning the treatment being offered, including potential hazards and risks. This duty and legal principal that a mentally competent adult has control over his or her own body requires a physician to obtain the patient's informed consent before beginning medical treatment.

Informed consent will develop from the patient's understanding of the following factors:

- General nature of the treatment and consequences involved
- Normal risks and hazards of inherent treatment
- Side effects or complications known to occur
- Alternative treatments

FRAUD AND ABUSE

Any medical practice treating Medicare patients must be aware of the strict fraud and abuse rules governing Medicare billing. The Office of Inspector General (OIG) is responsible for identifying and eliminating fraud and abuse. The OIG carries out this mission through a nationwide network of audits, investigations, and inspections of physician's offices.

The most common inspection by the OIG is the Medicare audit to identify inconsistencies in billing, coverage, and payment of bills for particular services.

The Centers for Medicare and Medicaid Services (CMS) defines Medicare fraud as "knowingly and willfully making or causing a false statement or representation of a material fact made in application for a Medicare benefit of payment." Fraud occurs when a physician knowingly bills Medicare for a service that was not rendered or when the physician overstates or exaggerates a particular service.

Some examples of Medicare fraud are as follows:

- An indication that there may be deliberate application of duplicate reimbursement
- Any false representation with respect to the nature of charges for services rendered

- A claim for uncovered services billed as services that are covered
- A claim involving collusion between the physician and recipient resulting in higher costs or charges

Medicare abuse refers to activities that may directly or indirectly cause financial losses to the Medicare program or the beneficiary. Abuse generally occurs when the physician operates in a manner that is inconsistent with accepted business and medical practices.

The most common types of abuse are:

- The overuse of medical services (eg, repeated lab testing when results are normal, etc).
- Up-coding and overuse of office visits.
- Waiving copayments for patient's deductible portion. Physicians are required to collect the 20 percent Medicare co-payment from the Medicare patient. Routinely waiving the co-payment, unless in very unusual cases, such as extreme financial hardship, is considered a fraudulent activity.

THE MEDICAL RECORD

A well-documented, legible, structured medical record is the physician's first line of defense if there is a malpractice suit. The medical record is a form of communication among health care professionals about the patient's condition. This documentation identifies the patient, supports the diagnosis, justifies the treatment, and documents the results of treatment.

The medical record is confidential. The information is private; it should remain secure and not made public. While the record belongs to the physician, the information belongs to the patient.

Authorization to Release Records

Sole authority to release information from the medical record belongs to the patient. The office should be prepared with a printed release form that the patient signs to release the medical record to a third party. The release form need not be complicated or full of legal language.

As a word of caution, HIV/AIDS information is *not* included in a standard release form. The release form must *specifically* state that the release includes this information. Any mention of HIV/AIDS testing or treatment is extremely sensitive and should be maintained in a separate part of the medical record. Some attorneys suggest it should be maintained in an envelope marked, *CONFIDENTIAL! DO NOT RELEASE.*

Records are the heart of systematic patient care. Excellent record keeping is one of the most effective tools in patient care and in preventing claims. Following are the key elements of a good medical record:

- **Uniform Records.** Medical records should be uniform within the practice. An excellent way to structure charts is to insert dividers for lab, x-ray, progress notes, etc, and to use a problem list. In this format, the record is organized for easy scanning by all health care professionals who subsequently use the chart.

- **Secure Pages.** Secure all pages of the record in chronological order with fasteners to prevent pages from being lost.

- **Organization.** Organize records for easy and accurate retrieval. Whatever system is used, it should be logical and clear to all staff members and physicians (eg, active versus inactive patients, color coding for chronic problems or frequent diagnoses, etc).

- **Timeliness.** Make all entries in the record, whether written or dictated, at the time of the patient contact. Include the date and the time of the exam or contact. The greater the time lapse between the exam and the entry, the less credible the medical record becomes.

- **Legible Records.** Records must be legible. Health care professionals with illegible handwriting should dictate their notes or use electronic medical records (EMR). This helps to avoid misinterpretations that result in improper treatment.

- **Dictated Records.** Dictated notes must be proofread and signed. The statement *"dictated but not read"* does not relieve the physician from responsibility for what was transcribed. At best, the statement alerts another health care professional that the note has not been proofed and may not be correct.

- **Accurate Records.** Recording all information in objective and concise terms is important. Never include extraneous information, subjective assessments, or derogatory comments about the patient. Include direct quotations from the patient. Reduce the essential information to the least possible number of words.

- **Corrections.** Never improperly or unlawfully alter a medical record. Do not obliterate an entry with a marker or whiteout. If an error has been made, draw a single line through the inaccurate entry and enter the necessary correction. Date, time, and initial the correction in the margin. Making an addendum to a medical record is also acceptable. It should be made after the last entry noting the current date and time, and both entries should be cross-referenced. A record that appears to have been altered implies that a cover-up has occurred.

- **Jousting.** Never criticize or make derogatory comments about another health care professional or organization to the patient or in the medical record. A negative comment can undermine a patient's confidence in the previous health care worker and contribute to or cause a decision to pursue a legal claim regardless of causation and/or who was responsible.

- **Patient Telephone Calls.** Document all patient telephone calls in the medical record. When speaking to a patient while you are away from the office, and the medical record is not available, record notes on a call pad regarding any prescriptions or medical advice given over the telephone. The sheet can be presented for entry into the chart when you return to the office.

■ **Conversations.** Address and document all patient/family worries or concerns in the patient record. Record the source of the information, if other than the patient.

■ **Important Instructions.** Always document important warnings and instructions given to the patient at the time of discharge. Documenting discharge instructions may help prove a patient's noncompliance. Juries are less sympathetic toward noncompliant patients.

■ **Informed Consent.** To reinforce the signed informed consent form, always document information disclosed during the informed consent process.

■ **Potential Complications.** Document all possible complications that might occur. Failure to recognize a complication in time to prevent injury is a common basis for a lawsuit. Proving negligence is difficult if the record shows prior awareness that a complication might occur.

Medical Records Documentation

A great deal of emphasis has been placed recently on the thorough documentation of patient encounters. Not only is documentation critical to reduce the possibility of malpractice, it is also a necessity in claiming proper reimbursement.

Many physicians have been unsuccessful in defending malpractice suits due to incomplete or illegible medical records. Malpractice insurance carriers and risk management experts recommend the following tips as loss prevention initiatives:

■ Fasten all materials into the chart.

■ Dictate progress notes and have them transcribed, if possible.

■ Clearly identify allergies on the chart.

■ Enter the patient's name on every page in the chart.

■ The physician should initial every entry in the medical record.

■ Financial data should not be kept in the chart.

Figure 14-2 is a sample of a medical records checklist form that can be used when checking a patient's chart. To minimize risk, check 10 to 20 charts periodically to assure that these guidelines are being met.

Documentation to Support Level of Service

Most Managed Care Organizations (MCOs) have definite guidelines for documenting patient encounters. Sometimes they conduct post-payment audits in the physician's office to assure that the documentation on the patient's medical chart supports the service that was charged, and to assure that the physician took the proper steps to reach a satisfactory diagnosis. Medicare also conducts post-payment audits and will usually request that the physician mail in

FIGURE 14-2

Medical Records Checklist Form

MEDICAL RECORDS CHECKLIST			
	Yes	**No**	**N/A**
Patient name on all pages			
All pages secured with fasteners			
Forms organized with tabs for easy access			
Organized chronologically			
Legible entries			
Missed appoints documented			
Telephone message documented			
Allergies uniformly documented			
Entries dated, timed, and initialed			
Dictation proofread and initialed			
Only standard abbreviations used			
Diagnostic reports initialed prior to filing			
Reason for visit documented			
Clinical findings (positive/negative) documented			
Treatment plan documented			
Entries are objective			
Patient instructions documented			
Patient education materials given/documented			
Medication List			
1. Current			
2. Prescriptions			
3. Refills			
4. Allergies			
Informed consent on chart			
Consultation reports on chart			
Problem list kept current			

photocopies of specific patient records. Both MCOs and Medicare will require the physician to repay any amount paid for a service that is not supported by proper documentation. These repayments can sometimes amount to thousands of dollars.

To avoid this type of risk, begin during the start-up phase to set up the patient records according to the guidelines in this chapter, and make thorough documentation as convenient and efficient as possible. Existing charts (inherited from other practitioners) can be converted over time and information organized for efficiency. Preprinted forms are recommended for progress notes, medication records, telephone calls, and other reports.

Charting the Patient's Progress

Using a standard format to record the patient's visit will assure that every encounter includes all the components that are necessary for complete documentation. The American Academy of Family Practice recommends the SOAP format. Utilizing the SOAP format, the physician records the patient encounter as follows:

S = Subjective findings

O = Objective findings

A = Assessment of problem/complaint

P = Plan of treatment

This format is easily followed by any health care provider and should be complete if the record is ever subpoenaed in a legal case.

ORGANIZING THE PATIENT FILE

Having every patient's chart organized in the same order saves time. It takes less time to locate a specific report or item the physician needs to properly treat the patient.

Figure 14-3 is an example of how a patient's chart might be organized for greater efficiency.

FIGURE 14-3

Sample Patient's Chart Map

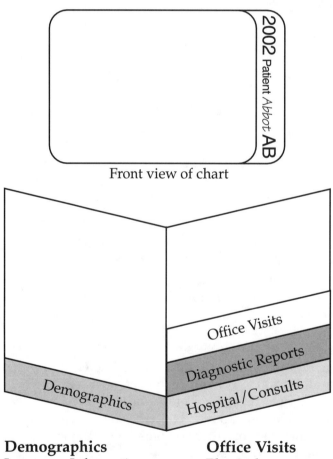

Front view of chart

Demographics
Insurance Information
Insurance/Correspondence
 Divider
Correspondence

Office Visits
Physicals
Medication Reports

Diagnostic Reports
Lab Reports
X-Ray Reports
All Other Diagnostic Reports

Hospital/Consults

CONCLUSION

Risk management is vital to the success of your practice. Be mindful of your liabilities in every aspect of your practice. In addition to having the proper insurance coverage for your liabilities, be sure to have the proper procedures and protocols in place to make a difference in your exposure to risk.

REFERENCE

Dunevitz B. Risk management program can mean the difference between success and legal failure. *MGM Update*. 2000; 39. http://www2.mgma.com/literature/?MIval=full_text&ID=11244&sub=MGM+Update&syear=. 09/06/02.

chapter 15

Building Your Practice Through Marketing

INTRODUCTION

A rapidly changing health care environment is constantly challenging physicians to adopt strategies to attract new patients and maintain the loyalties of existing patients. If the term *marketing* is a concern and it contains negative connotations, think of these strategies as building or expanding the practice. Whatever the description, these actions are a vital part of your success.

DEVELOPING MARKETING STRATEGIES

The strategies that are employed to attract new patients are generally very tangible, such as the Yellow Pages or newspaper advertisements, or even a website on the Internet. These are called external marketing strategies. Internal strategies are directed toward retaining the patient base and increasing loyalty through subliminal activities. The physician and staff accomplish these through friendliness and efficiency, expressed by communication and concern. This chapter provides some suggestions on both internal and external marketing strategies.

The Marketing Budget

As the first year's operational budget is established, include a specific amount for marketing expenses. Establishing a marketing budget is an extremely important step in the development of the practice's promotional efforts. There are many ways to advance your practice, and every method has its costs. Do not consider these expenditures as optional; they are as vital to your success as having the proper equipment. If you do not expend the necessary time and money, you may suffer the consequences in loss of patients to the competition.

Obtain quotes on the development and printing of a practice brochure, appointment and business cards, letterhead, other stationery, and educational materials. Factor these costs into the first year's budget and include the costs of any other marketing expense you might have such as a newspaper announcement and a Yellow Pages listing.

The Marketing Plan

Just as you have planned for the furniture and equipment needs in starting your practice, you will want to establish a marketing plan. The plan need not be complicated or formal, but it is imperative that it is committed to paper. Share this plan with your staff. They will become an integral part of your marketing efforts.

Four months before opening:

■ Check sources such as *The Welcome Wagon* and groups that present information to new residents. Supply handout items for their distribution.

■ Set up a system to track how patients are referred to the practice. One method is to use a referral log, a simple grid that lists the various sources of referral. Referrals come from various sources (eg, the newspaper, Yellow Pages, a presentation made at a civic group, another physician or patient, etc). Always ask patients the name of the patient, physician, or other individual who referred them to you. Send a note to that person saying, "Thank you for the referral."

■ Attend meetings and join civic groups that will enhance your presence in the community. If you have children in the local school system, join the Parent-Teachers Association. Offer to speak to these organizations on medical topics. Tell the Medical Staff Secretary at your hospital(s) that you are available for public speaking engagements.

■ Check with local hospitals to see if these institutions have planned health fairs or health screenings in the future. Offer to participate.

Three months before opening:

■ Develop a practice brochure. An attractive, well-prepared brochure provides your patients with all the information they need about the practice. Include a short paragraph about yourself, your specialty, and your education. Add a photograph for a good touch. If the budget does not permit a professionally prepared brochure, use computer software and a laser printer to print information about your practice. (See *Brochure Contents* section at the end of this chapter for an outline of a practice brochure.)

Two months before opening:

■ Design and place an order for announcement cards to send to local physicians and other health care professionals. These announcements should show your name, specialty, address, and telephone number; mail at least two weeks before opening.

■ Order stationery and appointment cards with the letterhead and logo if one has been developed. Order only small amounts to begin. Changes may need to be made later.

One month before opening:

■ Order patient education materials for the practice. Use a rubber stamp to imprint your name and address on the front of every piece of educational information that is handed out or placed in the waiting room. This information may find its way to another potential patient.

- Visit the Hospital(s) where you will be on staff. Introduce yourself to the department heads and nursing staff.

- If you are providing treatment for work injuries, rehabilitation, or other occupationally related services, visit the employers in the area; introduce yourself and the services you provide. Take copies of your practice brochure and your business cards. Meet with the person responsible for Workers' Compensation injuries or treatment, and the benefits coordinator.

   Two weeks before opening day:

- Draft a newspaper advertisement and submit it to the local newspaper(s). The advertisement should give your name, address, and telephone number. It should define and briefly describe your specialty and services that will be offered. Also, indicate the hours of operation.

- Meet with your staff to share the marketing plan and ask for ideas. Patients who call for an appointment will want to know a little about you. Give each employee a copy of your Curriculum Vitae and outline your specialty training. Tell them about yourself so they can discuss your credentials with potential patients. Explaining to your staff the types of services provided by your specialty is also helpful. Keep in mind that your staff is *marketing* the practice's services to patients as well.

- Conduct office staff training on telephone communications to patients and referring physicians. If you receive a referral from a physician you have not previously met, it is a good idea to speak to that physician yourself. Put these protocols in writing and make them a part of the Policies and Procedures Manual. Tell your staff how much time is needed for specific types of appointments. Allow extra time for any first visit; you will be building relationships during this time.

PRACTICE BUILDING GUIDELINES FOR THE FUTURE

With any marketing effort, developing guidelines is important. Clarify your thoughts and plans on paper and follow these suggestions:

- **Define your objectives.** Define these for the short-term (less than one year); then define them for the long-term (more than one year). Express them in a way that they can be quantified and tracked so that successes and failures can be measured.

- **Caution!** Practically all professionals automatically say, "I'd like to double my practice." It is not as simple as that. Determine how much time and energy can be spent to achieve that goal. To play conservatively, figure that the budget must amount to 20 percent to 33 percent of the targeted increase in income to generate an equally conservative 333 percent to 500 percent.

- **Remember cash flow.** Many strategies call for 50 percent to 75 percent of the marketing budget to be spent in the first 25 percent of the time. This usually means that the first large sum of cash needs to be in the bank at the start of the program, so it cannot come out of unexpected cash flow.

- **Identify the target groups.** Define the groups that the practice is trying to reach. Describe the target populations by the chief characteristics of age, sex, location, educational level, income, ethnicity/religion, blue-collar workers versus white-collar workers, and lifestyle. Choose only those factors that are most important, usually income, education, sex, age, and location. If business is targeted, describe it by industry, industry position, yearly sales, number of employees, and location.

- **Create a different, one-page marketing plan for each target.** For example, set up a plan for other practitioners from whom to generate referrals, senior citizens, blue-collar workers, 18- to 34-year-old females, and so on. Then rank those groups, targeting the easiest first.

- **Define what the target groups want.** What are the characteristics most important to the target group in selecting a physician in that specific field? Is it experience, hours, location, price?

- **Define the physician.** Strengths? Weaknesses? What is different or special about the physician concerning his or her education, expertise, years of experience, credentials? What does the practice offer in terms of location, hours, pricing, and special equipment?

- **Analyze the main competitors.** Analyze just the competitors with whom the practice will compete in the service area. Do not ignore the indirect competitors outside the profession to whom prospects could turn as a substitute, such as chiropractors, podiatrists, or psychologists. Chart each competitor's strengths and weaknesses.

- **How to compete.** How does the practice rate against those main competitors? Where can the practice best compete? List primary points. Then secondary points. Can the targets be serviced well, or is the practice going too far outside its area of expertise? Assume the physician has good, solid experience, but that a competitor has more. If that competitor does not promote experience and the practice does, the practice will have the reputation for experience with the public. The same is true for any other advantage.

- **Determine the budget.** How much can the practice afford now? Reconcile the budget with the goals.

- **Choose a strategy.** Should it be internal promotion? Yellow Pages? Newspapers? Public relations? Seminars? Is this strategy the most effective one? Weigh the pros and cons of various vehicles against each other.

- **Choose the timing.** List events, both external and internal, that will affect the campaign over the period that has been specified.

Choose the time of year, which months, and what week to take action. If the practice has seasonal peaks, promote heavily upon entering those busier periods, not during the practice lows. Dollars and efforts must work a lot harder in low periods when prospects are not already looking for services.

- **Plan the execution.** Assign responsibilities. Set deadlines for all steps on a master time line.

BUILDING PATIENT SATISFACTION

In a pure fee-for-service market, a patient's dissatisfaction with a physician generally amounts to the loss of that one patient and possibly the loss of another family member. In a market dominated by managed care organizations, patient dissatisfaction can result in the loss of an entire patient population.

Managed Care Organizations gather a tremendous amount of data from their enrollees and use this information as a component in grading the plan's physicians. If a physician fails to make the grade, he or she may be dropped from the plan.

Be proactive in attempts to increase patient satisfaction. After the practice has been established about six months, conduct a patient satisfaction survey. Survey at least 100 patients or, if possible, every patient. Invaluable opinions about the practice, the staff, and the physician's own success up to this point can be gained. Take the patients' suggestions seriously. Carry out any changes that will increase patient satisfaction. Figure 15-1 is a sample patient satisfaction survey.

Practice Services and Amenities

Marketing can be as simple as making every patient feel comfortable and appreciated. Differentiate the practice from others by providing a personal touch to patient relationships. Follow these guidelines as a part of the practice's approach to patient service:

- Assign someone in the office the responsibility of managing the practice's relationships with its most important customers.
- Send a welcome letter to a patient after they have made the initial appointment. Thank the patient and enclose a practice brochure.
- Acknowledge patients immediately upon arrival.
- Always address a patient by name. Be very sensitive to the patient's feelings in deciding whether to use formal or informal terms of address.
- Explain all lengthy delays, and make sure that patients are given the opportunity to reschedule if they so desire. The physician(s) should be encouraged to be punctual and attentive to the appointment schedule. Remember, the patient's time is valuable, too!

FIGURE 15-1

Patient Satisfaction Survey

	YES	NO
Do you feel you understand the specialty of our practice?	☐	☐
Do you believe you are aware of all the services we offer?	☐	☐
Is the location of our office convenient?	☐	☐
Do you find our waiting room comfortable?	☐	☐
Do you feel relaxed in the waiting room?	☐	☐
Are our parking facilities adequate?	☐	☐
Do you have to pay to park when you come to see us?	☐	☐
If yes, is this a hindrance to receiving your care here?	☐	☐
Do you have to pay to park when you see other practitioners?	☐	☐
What change would you make in the physician aspects of our office?	☐	☐
Do you find our front office personnel (eg, secretary) friendly and courteous?	☐	☐
Do you find our business personnel (eg, practice manager, bookkeeper) friendly and courteous?	☐	☐
Are your telephone calls handled in a prompt, courteous manner?	☐	☐
Are you receiving adequate help with your insurance?	☐	☐
Have you received a copy of our business policies?	☐	☐
Have our payment and billing policies been explained to your satisfaction?	☐	☐
Do you find our nurses friendly and courteous?	☐	☐
Do you feel our nurses are sympathetic to your illness?	☐	☐
Do you find the doctor(s) friendly?	☐	☐
Do you feel the doctor is interested in you as a person?	☐	☐
Does the doctor spend enough time with you?	☐	☐
Is your wait too long in the reception area before you see the doctor?	☐	☐
Do you have to wait too long in the examination room before you see the doctor?	☐	☐
Is our answering service prompt and courteous?	☐	☐
Do our doctors promptly return your calls?	☐	☐
Are your telephone calls to the doctors during the day?	☐	☐
Do you mind if the nurses respond to some of your calls?	☐	☐
Are you satisfied with the hospital we use?	☐	☐
Is this hospital convenient for you and your family?	☐	☐
Do you feel that our fees are high?	☐	☐
Average?	☐	☐
Have you used other health services (such as an emergency clinic) because you felt it would be less expensive? If yes, which one(s)? _____	☐	☐
Do you have trouble getting an appointment when you would like?	☐	☐
Are our secretaries helpful in finding appointments that meet your needs?	☐	☐
Are our office hours convenient for you?	☐	☐
If not, how could we better serve you? _____		
Would you like more educational information from us?	☐	☐
If we have audiovisual tapes available about your medical problem, would you use them?	☐	☐

Figure 15-1 *Continued*

Patient Satisfaction Survey

	YES	NO
Would you want to receive a health newsletter from us periodically?	☐	☐
How were you referred to this practice?		
☐ Other patients ☐ Friends ☐ Yellow Pages ☐ Medical Society ☐ Another doctor ☐ Our reputation ☐ Other: _____		
Are you satisfied enough with the care we provide to refer other people to us?	☐	☐

- Let patients with disabilities or the elderly know that pre-arrangement can be made for a staff member to meet them at their car to be escorted into the office. Have a wheelchair available.

- Provide educational materials; they usually help patients become more able and willing to assume responsibility in assisting in the healing process. Many forms are commercially available or the practice can write its own educational materials, produce videos or audio cassettes, and establish a lending library.

- Ask about the patient's family. Some physicians jot down personal notes about each patient and keep them in the patient's chart. Some physicians even have photographs taken of each patient and attach them to charts to refresh their memory.

- Spend adequate time with each patient. Surveys show that patient satisfaction directly correlates with how much time the physician spends with the patient.

- Create a pleasant reception area:
  - Provide a living room effect
  - Decorate tastefully
  - Use table lamps rather than fluorescent lighting
  - Display arrangements of fresh cut flowers
  - Provide educational videos on interesting health topics
  - Provide tasteful distractions, such as an aquarium, art objects, wall hangings
  - Play soothing, easy-listening music
  - Offer patients something to do (eg, puzzles, books, crossword puzzles, current magazines)

Standards of Patient Service for Medical Staff

Each member of the staff should render services to patients with the highest professional standards. The following guidelines serve as effective reminders of how best to treat patients:

- Acknowledge patients promptly and courteously with eye contact and a pleasant expression and tone of voice.

- When talking with patients and/or other employees, use words that express respect, patience, and understanding.

- Care for people with kindness and gentleness, rather than with cold professionalism.
- Address adult patients by their proper title and last name, unless the patient requests otherwise.
- Display visible identification and introduce yourself by name and title when first meeting a patient.
- Answer the telephone quickly and courteously; identify yourself by name. Provide callers the opportunity to respond to a request to be placed on hold, and explain to them if their call is being transferred.
- Be sensitive to reducing noise levels near patient care areas.
- Respect patient privacy by knocking before entering the room if the door is closed, and by refraining from discussing one patient in front of another.
- Protect the confidentiality of patients, coworkers, and others who use the facilities.
- Make certain that patient modesty is always respected.
- Be attentive to patients and their families who are kept waiting in waiting areas or treatment rooms for extended periods.
- Consider the effect of what is said and done in the presence of patients. Refrain from conducting personal (not work-related) conversations in front of patients.
- Refrain from discussing other employees, organizational policies, problems, or medical care in public areas.
- Maintain and use medical equipment and facilities appropriately and cost-effectively.

YELLOW PAGES ADVERTISING

A well-designed Yellow Pages advertisement can work for the practice 24 hours a day, 365 days a year. Statistics suggest that practices attract 5 percent to 10 percent of their new patients through Yellow Pages advertising. They are also useful for attracting patients who have not been to the practice for some time.

Before placing an ad, evaluate what other colleagues are doing. Then look through the Yellow Pages from another community and compare styles, design, size, and text. What makes the ad stand out from the rest? Which ads are more attractive?

The goal is to make the practice's ad unique and to grab the shopper's attention. Achieving this without discrediting the practice with a cluttered distasteful ad is very important. A simple, clean, and professionally designed ad that is 2" × 3" can be very effective. The following checklist will help the practice create an effective, powerful, and attractive ad.

- Is the practice's name, specialty, and telephone number the most prominent elements in the ad?
- Has the name of the practice been included with the name(s) of the physician(s) in the practice?

- Have any special qualifications such as board certification been included?
- Are area locators, such as cross streets or building names, mentioned with the listing of the office address?
- Have all extended hours been listed?
- Have all special services been included?
- If the practice has a logo or slogan, was it included in the ad?
- Have the ad sizes for competitors been reviewed to determine an appropriate-sized ad for the practice?
- Should boldface type be used to call attention to the ad?
- Does the chosen typeface correspond to the character of the practice?
- Does the ad reflect the image that the practice hopes to project?

CREATING A MEDICAL PRACTICE BROCHURE

A practice brochure creates many marketing opportunities. It creates an image of the practice to current and prospective patients and referral sources. The brochure provides information about available services, office policies, and practice philosophy. It also saves the staff's time by addressing repetitive questions, such as where the physician has hospital privileges or how insurance is billed. The brochure will serve as a compact reference about the practice.

How to Create a Brochure

The best resources for creating a brochure are colleagues and other professional businesses. To obtain ideas, collect samples of attractive brochures. A typical brochure has six to eight panels of information and is 3 1/2″ × 8 1/2″. Write the copy or hire a professional to help with the writing. The goal of the brochure is to clarify practice policies, written in language that is clear and concise.

Brochure Contents

The practice brochure should contain the following information:

- **Introduction to the practice.** Begin by including the name, address, and telephone number of the practice. Provide a brief history of the practice and state the patient care and philosophy.
- **Professional profile of the physician(s).** Introduce each physician in the practice and include details on training, board certification, areas of special interest, and personal information. For example, "Dr Doe is married and has two school-aged children," or "Dr Smith enjoys working in underserved countries one month each year." Include a picture of each physician to help patients with name and face recognition.
- **Explanation of specialty.** Quite frequently, physicians and their staffs are not aware that patients do not know or understand a

physician's specialty and the part of the anatomy to which it pertains. They assume that once a patient gets as far as the reception room, the patient has a thorough understanding of why he or she is there. To educate the patient about the practice, include a description, in simple terms, of the practice specialty and the special services and procedures that can be provided. The more informed a patient is before the visit, the more confidence he or she has in the care that is received.

- **Office policies.** One primary objective of a practice brochure is to educate and inform patients about practice policies. It serves as a reference and reminder to established patients and provides guidelines and standards for new patients before incurring services.

Key areas to highlight include:

- **Office hours.** This is especially critical if appointment times are beyond the typical practice hours (ie, evening, Saturday hours). Stating office hours will also reduce after-hours calls to the answering service and consequently reduce overhead expenses.

- **How to schedule and cancel appointments.** If patients are asked to use a different telephone number for scheduling appointments, publicize it. If there are a lot of no-show patients, it is very important to establish and state the policy that will discourage this abuse and encourage compliance. Charging $25 for a no-show or a late cancellation is customary for practices (within 24 hours of scheduled appointment). If a patient abuses either policy three times, he or she should receive a letter discharging him or her from care within a reasonable period (ie, 30 days). To protect the practice, send the letter via certified mail, return receipt requested. (See the Sample Discharge Letter in Chapter 14, *Loss Prevention and Risk Management.*)

- **Hospital affiliations.** The insurance industry may influence a patient's selection of both a hospital and a physician. Therefore, including hospital affiliations in the practice brochure is important.

- **Financial policies.** Generally, the most frequently asked questions pertain to the practice's financial policies. Document these policies in the brochure to inform patients about their financial responsibility.

Include the forms of accepted payment (ie, cash, check, credit card). Most practices follow the policy that they expect payment when they render services unless the patient makes other arrangements. This policy should be stated.

Identify the insurance plans in which the practice participates (eg, IPA, PPO, HMO). Also state whether or not the practice accepts Medicare assignment. Include billing information, such as when the patient should expect to receive a statement, after what period an account will be placed in collection, and so forth. Be sure to include the telephone number to call regarding billing questions.

- **Special services.** Health care consumers will look for practices that offer one-stop shopping. List all services that the practice offers, such as laboratory and radiology services. Also list special procedures or testing that is offered (eg, infertility tests, nutrition counseling, pain management).

- **Telephone calls.** If the practice has an established office policy regarding prescription refills, print it in the brochure. Patients need to know how to handle routine prescription refills. Informing them of the policy makes the office more efficient and responsive to the patient's request.

Notifying patients that an answering service will respond to calls after normal office hours is important. Patients appreciate knowing a voice is always on the other end of the line, and that the physician will get their message. Consider printing the answering service telephone number for the rare occasion the office forgets to sign off to the service after hours. Printing the physician's pager number is not advisable.

- **Map of office location.** Including a map of the office location is as important as printing the name and telephone number of the practice. The map should include landmarks, such as a hospital, a lake, a park, or something with which the patient may be familiar. If the office is close to the hospital, it adds a competitive marketing edge. It is to the physician's benefit to include this information.

CONCLUSION

Building a medical practice takes a concerted effort and careful planning. Typically, in the early stages of practice start-up, marketing funds are limited. Be sure to spend all marketing dollars wisely and appropriately in the area and specialty. If help is needed, get assistance from a reliable and experienced health care consultant who can keep the practice focused on initiatives that are most likely to be beneficial.

Professional Associations

American Academy of Family Physicians
11400 Tomahawk Creek Parkway
Leawood, KS 66211-2672
Telephone: (913) 906-6000
E-mail: fp@aafp.org
http://www.aafp.org

American College of Obstetricians and Gynecologists
409 12th Street, SW, P.O. Box 96920
Washington, DC 20090-6920
http://www.acog.com/

The American Academy of Pediatrics
141 Northwest Point Boulevard
Elk Grove Village, IL 60007-1098
Telephone: (847) 434-4000
Fax: (847) 434-8000
http://www.aap.org/

American Academy of Otolaryngology-Head and Neck Surgery
One Prince St.
Alexandria, VA 22314-3357
Telephone: (703) 836-4444
http://www.entnet.org/

The American College of Cardiology
Heart House
9111 Old Georgetown Road
Bethesda, MD 20814-1699
Telephone: (800) 253-4636, ext. 694 or (301) 897-5400
Fax: (301) 897-9745
http://www.acc.org/

American Academy of Neurology
1080 Montreal Avenue
St. Paul, MN 55116
Telephone: (651) 695-1940
http://www.aan.com/

American Academy of Ophthalmology
P.O. Box 7424
San Francisco, CA 94120
Telephone: (415) 561-8500
http://www.aao.org/

American College of Surgeons
633 N. Saint Clair Street
Chicago, IL 60611-3211
Telephone: (312) 202-5000
Fax: (312) 202-5001
E-mail: postmaster@facs.org
http://www.facs.org/

American Urological Association
1120 North Charles Street
Baltimore, MD 21201
Telephone: (410) 727-1100
Fax: (410) 223-4370
http://www.auanet.org/

American Academy of Orthopaedic Surgeons
6300 North River Road
Rosemont, IL 60018-4262
Telephone: (847) 823-7186 or (800) 356-AAOS
Fax: (847) 823-8125
AAOS Fax on Demand: (800) 999-2939
http://www.aaos.org/

American Association of Neurological Surgeons
5550 Meadowbrook Drive
Rolling Meadows, IL 60088
Telephone: (847) 378-0500 or (888) 566-AANS (2267)
Fax: (847) 378-0600
E-mail: info@aans.org
http://www.neurosurgery.org/aans/

American Psychiatric Association
1400 K Street, NW
Washington, DC 20005
Telephone: (888) 357-7924
Fax: (202) 682-6850
E-mail: apa@psych.org
http://www.psych.org/

Renal Physicians Association
4701 Randolph Road, Suite 102
Rockville, MD 20852
Telephone: (301) 468-3515
Fax: (301) 468-3511
http://www.renalmd.org/

American Academy of Physical Medicine and Rehabilitation
One IBM Plaza, Suite 2500
Chicago, IL 60611-3604
Telephone: (312) 464-9700
Fax: (312) 464-0227
E-mail: info@aapmr.org
http://www.aapmr.org/

American Academy of Physician Assistants
950 North Washington Street
Alexandria, VA 22314-1552
Telephone: (703) 836-2272
Fax: (703) 684-1924
http://www.aapa.org/

American Academy of Nurse Practitioners
P.O. Box 12846
Austin, TX 78711
Telephone: (512) 442-4262
Fax: (512) 442-6469
E-mail: admin@aanp.org
http://www.aanp.org/

American Academy of Allergy, Asthma & Immunology
611 East Wells Street
Milwaukee, WI 53202
Telephone: (414) 272-6071
Patient Information and Physician Referral Line: 1 (800) 822-2762
http://www.aaaai.org/

The American Academy of Child and Adolescent Psychiatry
3615 Wisconsin Avenue, NW
Washington, DC 20016-3007
Telephone: (202) 966-7300
Fax: (202) 966-2891
http://www.aacap.org/

The American Academy of Dermatology
930 E. Woodfield Road
Schaumburg, IL 60173-4927
Telephone: (847) 330-0230
Fax: (847) 330-0050
http://www.aad.org/

American Academy of Facial Plastic and Reconstructive Surgery
310 S. Henry Street
Alexandria, VA 22314
Telephone: (703) 299-9291
Fax: (703) 299-8898
http://www.facial-plastic-surgery.org/

American Academy of Insurance Medicine
5701 Golden Hills Drive
Minneapolis, MN 55416-1297
Telephone: (763) 765-6533
Fax: (763) 765-6520
http://www.aaimedicine.org/

American Academy of Pain Medicine
4700 W. Lake
Glenview, IL 60025
Telephone: (847) 375-4731
Fax: (877) 734-8750
E-mail: aapm@amctec.com
http://www.painmed.org/

American Academy of Sleep Medicine
6301 Bandel Road, NW, Suite 101
Rochester, MN 55901
Telephone: (507) 287-6006
Fax: (507) 287-6008
http://www.aasmnet.org/

The American Association for Thoracic Surgery
Thirteen Elm Street
Manchester, MA 01944
Telephone: (978) 526-8330
Fax: (978) 526-7521
E-mail: aats@prri.com
http://www.aats.org/

American Association of Clinical Endocrinologists
1000 Riverside Avenue, Suite 205
Jacksonville, FL 32204
Telephone: (904) 353-7878
Fax: (904) 353-8185
http://www.aace.com/

American Association of Public Health Physicians
AAPHP PMB #1720, P.O. Box 2430
Pensacola, FL 32513-2430
http://www.aaphp.org/

American College of Chest Physicians
3300 Dundee Road
Northbrook, IL 60062-2348
Telephone: (847) 498-1400
Fax: (847) 498-5460
E-mail: accp@chestnet.org
http://www.chestnet.org/

American College of Emergency Physicians
1125 Executive Circle
Irving, TX 75038-2522
Telephone: (800) 798-1822
http://www.acep.org/

American College of Gastroenterology
4900 B South 31st Street
Arlington, VA 22206-1656
Telephone: (703) 820-7400
Fax: (703) 931-4520
http://www.acg.gi.org/

American Gastroenterological Association
National Office
7910 Woodmont Avenue, Suite 700
Bethesda, MD 20814
Telephone: (301) 654-2055
Fax: (301) 654-5920
http://www.gastro.org/

American College of Medical Quality
4334 Montgomery Avenue
Bethesda, MD 20814
Telephone: (301) 913-9149 or (800) 924-2149
Fax: (301) 913-9142
http://www.acmq.org/

American College of Occupational and Environmental Medicine
1114 N. Arlington Heights Road
Arlington Heights, IL 60004-4770
Telephone: (847) 818-1800
Fax: (847) 818-9266
http://www.acoem.org/

American College of Physicians—American Society of Internal
    Medicine
190 N. Independence Mall West
Philadelphia, PA 19106-1572
Telephone: (800) 523-1546, x2600 or (215) 351-2600
http://www.acponline.org/

American College of Physician Executives
4890 West Kennedy Boulevard
Tampa, FL 33609
Telephone: (800) 562-8088
Fax: (813) 287-8993
http://www.acpe.org/

American College of Preventive Medicine
1307 New York Avenue, NW, Suite 200
Washington, DC 20005
Telephone: (202) 466-2044
Fax: (202) 466-2662
http://www.acpm.org/

American College of Radiation Oncology
820 Jorie Boulevard
Oak Brook, IL 60523
Telephone: (630) 368-3733
Fax: (630) 571-7837
http://www.acro.org/

American College of Radiology
1891 Preston White Drive
Reston, VA 20191-4397
Telephone: (800) 227-5463
http://www.acr.org/

American College of Rheumatology
1800 Century Place, Suite 250
Atlanta, GA 30345
Telephone: (404) 633-3777
Fax: (404) 633-1870
E-mail: acr@rheumatology.org
http://www.rheumatology.org/

American Geriatrics Society
The Empire State Building
350 Fifth Avenue, Suite 801
New York, NY 10118
Telephone: (212) 308-1414
Fax: (212) 832-8646
http://www.americangeriatrics.org/

American Orthopaedic Foot and Ankle Society
2517 Eastlake Avenue E
Seattle, WA 98102
Telephone: (206) 223-1120
Fax: (206) 223-1178
http://www.aofas.org/

American Roentgen Ray Society
44211 Slatestone Court
Leesburg, VA 20176-5109
Telephone: (703) 729-3353
Fax: (703) 729-4839
http://www.arrs.org/

American Society for Dermatologic Surgery
930 E. Woodfield Road
Schaumburg, IL 60173-4927
Telephone: (847) 330-9830
http://www.asds-net.org/

American Society for Gastrointestinal Endoscopy
13 Elm Street
Manchester, MA 01944-1314
Telephone: (978) 526-8330
Fax: (978) 526-4018
http://www.asge.org/

American Society for Reproductive Medicine
1209 Montgomery Highway
Birmingham, AL 35216-2809
Telephone: (205) 978-5000
Fax: (205) 978-5005
http://www.asrm.org/

American Society for Surgery of the Hand
6300 North River Road, Suite 600
Rosemont, IL 60018-4256
Telephone: (847) 384-8300
Fax: (847) 384-1435
E-mail: info@assh.org
http://www.hand-surg.org/

American Society for Therapeutic Radiology and Oncology
12500 Fair Lakes Circle, Suite 375
Fairfax, VA 22033-3882
Telephone: (703) 502-1550
Fax: (703) 502-7852
http://www.astro.org/

American Society of Abdominal Surgeons
675 Main Street
Melrose, MA 02176-3195
Telephone: (781) 665-6102
Fax: (781) 665-4127
http://www.gis.net/~absurg/

American Society of Addiction Medicine
4601 North Park Avenue, Arcade Suite 101
Chevy Chase, MD 20815
Telephone: (301) 656-3920
Fax: (301) 656-3815
E-mail: Email@asam.org
http://www.asam.org/

American Society of Anesthesiologists
520 N. Northwest Highway
Park Ridge, IL 60068-2573
Telephone: (847) 825-5586
Fax: (847) 825-1692
E-mail: mail@asahq.org
http://www.asahq.org/

The American Society of Bariatric Physicians
5453 East Evans Place
Denver, CO 80222-5234
Telephone: (303) 770-2526
Fax: (303) 779-4834
E-mail: bariatric@asbp.org
http://www.asbp.org/

American Society of Cataract and Refractive Surgery
4000 Legato Road, Suite 850
Fairfax, VA 22033
Telephone: (703) 591-2220
Fax: (703) 591-0614
http://www.ascrs.org/

American Society of Clinical Oncology
1900 Duke Street, Suite 200
Alexandria, VA 22314
Telephone: (703) 299-0150
Fax: (703) 299-1044
asco@asco.org
http://www.asco.org/

American Society for Clinical Pathology
2100 West Harrison Street
Chicago, IL 60612
Telephone: (312) 738-1336
E-mail: info@ascp.org
http://www.ascp.org/index.asp

American Society of Colon and Rectal Surgeons
85 W. Algonquin Road, Suite 550
Arlington Heights, IL 60005
Telephone: (847) 290-9184
Fax: (847) 290-9203
http://www.fascrs.org/ascrs-who.html

American Society of Hematology
1900 M Street, NW, Suite 200
Washington, DC 20036
Telephone: (202) 776-0544
Fax: (202) 776-0545
E-mail: ash@hematology.org
http://www.hematology.org/

American Society of Plastic Surgeons
Plastic Surgery Educational Foundation
444 E. Algonquin Road
Arlington Heights, IL 60005
Telephone: 1 (888) 4-PLASTIC—1 (888) 475-2784
http://www.plasticsurgery.org/

American Thoracic Society
1740 Broadway
New York, NY 10019-4374
Telephone: (212) 315-6440
Fax: (212) 315-6455
http://www.thoracic.org/

College of American Pathologists
325 Waukegan Road
Northfield, IL 60093
Telephone: (800) 323-4040
Fax: (847) 832-7000 in Illinois
http://www.cap.org/

The Endocrine Society
4350 East West Highway, Suite 500
Bethesda, MD 20814-4426
Telephone: (301) 941-0200
Fax: (301) 941-0259
E-mail: endostaff@endo-society.org
http://www.endo-society.org/

North American Spine Society
22 Calendar Court, 2nd Floor
LaGrange, IL 60525
Telephone: (877) Spine-Dr (toll free)
E-mail: info@spine.org
http://www.spine.org/

Radiological Society of North America, Inc.
820 Jorie Boulevard
Oak Brook, IL 60523-2251
Telephone: (630) 571-2670
Fax: (630) 571-7837
http://www.rsna.org/

Society of American Gastrointestinal Endoscopic Surgeons
2716 Ocean Park Boulevard, Suite 3000
Santa Monica, CA 90405
Telephone: (310) 314-2404
Fax: (310) 314-2585
http://www.sages.org/

Society of Cardiovascular & Interventional Radiology
10201 Lee Highway, Suite 500
Fairfax, VA 22030
Telephone: (800) 488-7284 or (703) 691-1805
Fax: (703) 691-1855
E-mail: info@scvir.org
http://www.scvir.org/

Society of Critical Care Medicine
701 Lee Street, Suite 200
Des Plaines, IL 60016
Telephone: (847) 827-6869
Fax: (847) 827-6886
E-mail: info@sccm.org
http://www.sccm.org/

Society of Nuclear Medicine
1850 Samuel Morse Drive
Reston, VA 20190-5316
Telephone: (703) 708-9000
Fax: (703) 708-9015
http://www.snm.org/

The Society of Thoracic Surgeons
401 North Michigan Avenue
Chicago, IL 60611-4267
Telephone: (312) 321-6803
Fax: (312) 527-6635
E-mail: sts@sba.com
http://www.sts.org/

Page numbers in *italics* represent figures or
 tables.

Are you taking advantage of these IBM resources available to you?

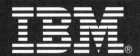

Ask the Experts.

Have a perplexing business or technical question? Our panel of independent small business experts may be able to help - at no cost to you! Send in your question, and ask the experts. Or search Frequently Asked Questions.

Small Business Advocate

Jim Blasingame and hundreds of small business experts share valuable information to maximize your business growth. Listen to his live or archived radio shows!

Go to **ibm.com**/smallbusiness/amalink

Small Business Owners tell it like it is...

See how business owners like yourself have grown their companies with the help of IBM technology. Our success stories speak for themselves!

IBM eNewsletter

Profit from e-business innovation. Every month, the IBM e-News for small business covers e-business strategies, e-commerce facts,testimonials, business stats and more!

visit **ibm.com**/smallbusiness/amalink

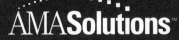

American Medical Association

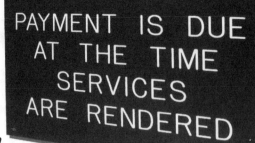
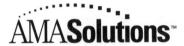
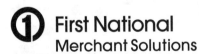

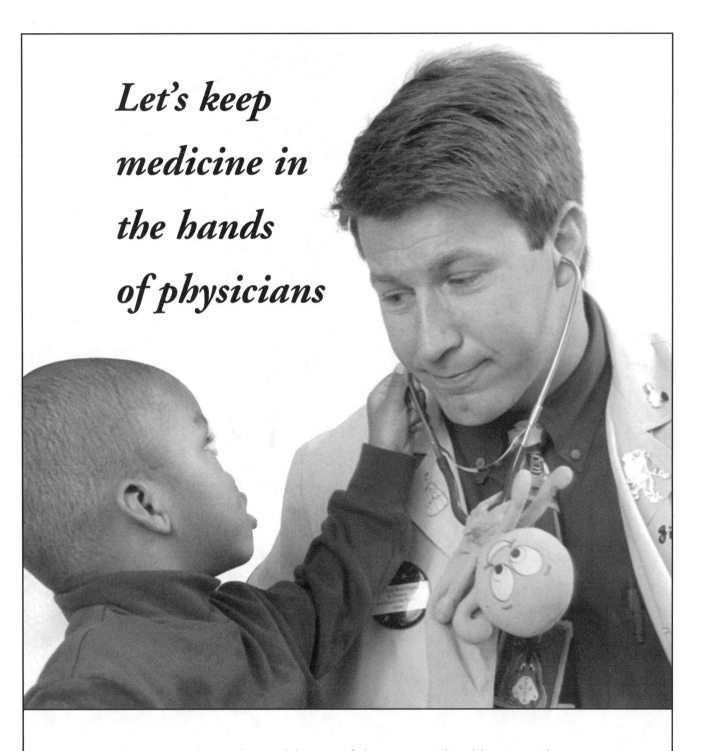

Let's keep medicine in the hands of physicians

Decisions about the well-being of the patient should not reside in the hands of administrators, legislators and lawyers. Protecting the physician-patient bond requires sustained, passionate and united efforts on the part of all physicians. Your involvement will determine the future health of America.

Be a member of the AMA.

800 262-3211 or visit *www.ama-assn.org*

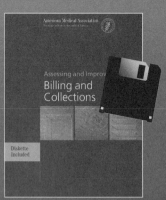
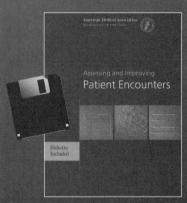
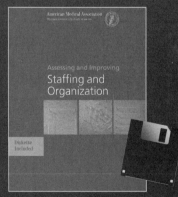

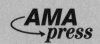